THE
KILLER PLAGUES
TO COME

THE KILLER PLAGUES TO COME

HOW YOU CAN BE INVULNERABLE TO THEM

William H. Lee, R.Ph., Ph.D.
Lynn Lee, CN

Instant Improvement, Inc.
New York

The intent of this book is solely informational and is in no way meant to be taken as nutritional or medical prescription. Please consult a health professional should the need for one be indicated.

Contents

PART I

The Killer Plagues To Come

Will Your Family Survive The Coming Fall of Antibiotics?

Yes — If You Start Anti-Germotic Home Treatment At Once!

Nature's Natural Germ Killers And Your Immune System Will Make The Difference Between Life or Death!

Foreword

WE BELIEVE that every newspaper, magazine and TV news program in this country should run the following headlines every single day:

DEADLY NEW PLAGUES INVADING AMERICA!

ANTIBIOTICS USELESS!

FLESH-EATING BACTERIA ARE ONLY THE BEGINNING!

MILLIONS MAY DIE AGONIZING DEATHS!

And, of course, we believe that our government should echo these warnings in every one of their publications and bulletins day in and day out.

Let's give you just one example: Thousands of hospital patients are dying TODAY from an untreatable new strain of staphylococcus bacteria. No antibiotic even slows it down. At present, it is confined to hospitals and infects only patients who have undergone transplants and bypasses. But in this group, it has reached runaway proportions.

When this killer spreads to the general population, doctors will weep in despair. But you will be safe.

This may be the greatest crisis yet faced by our human race. But there is still great hope. You can be among the few invulnerable survivors *if* you put to work the startling new discoveries inside these pages.

For these amazing new anti-germotics kill germs (both bacteria and viruses) that laugh at man-made antibiotics.

We would advise you to plague-proof your body and hoard these anti-germotics now. Take them every day of your life. Soon you may not be able to obtain them for any price.

Bill and Lynn Lee

Doctors will weep in despair. This may be the greatest crisis yet faced by our human race.

Chapter 1

Germ Warfare

NOT FROM Iraq or Iran.

Not from North Korea, Pakistan or any other first, second or third world country.

Germ Warfare from germs that have previously been thought to be of little consequence since the birth of antibiotic therapy.

What have we to fear? When your doctor says,

"I'm sorry. I just don't know what's happened. We've tried eight anti-biotics and nothing works. All that's left now is prayer."

You still have time to save yourself from hearing this, but barely enough.

Your great enemy is the jet plane. Every five minutes, jets are landing in this country from Africa, South America, China, the Mid-East and all the other great plague breeding grounds of the world.

No one checks these planes for bacteria. For viruses. For parasites. For invisible killers that have been born in swamps, in jungles, in hovels, in tiny villages all over the world where people sleep every night with animals that are covered with open infections.

And the terrifying fact is that, when one of these planes carries a new killer virus to our shores, it will produce 17 million offspring in the first 24 hours alone. It will be able to spread from person to person in a subway, or an office, or a school or a movie theater. By a handshake, or a cough, or a doorknob.

Are they on the next plane? Viruses that can tear apart the human heart? This crisis will engulf us all — not tomorrow — but today. Will your

"I'm sorry. I just don't know what's happened. We've tried eight antibiotics and nothing works. All that's left now is prayer."

*Soon,
all your doctor
will be able
to do
is wring
his hands
in despair.
All antibiotics
are
essentially
poisons
and the germs
have now
developed
armor plating
against those
poisons.*

immune system be capable of destroying a deadly virus hidden on a plane the moment it enters your body?

It will spread from the Pacific to the Atlantic in weeks. To every city and village and hamlet in America. No one anywhere will be safe.

And no antibiotic in medical science's exhausted arsenal will be able to slow down its deadly path because, every day, more and more antibiotics become useless.

Soon, all your doctor will be able to do is wring his hands in despair. Why?

Because all antibiotics are essentially poisons. And the germs have now developed armor plating against those poisons. Instead of the antibiotics killing them, now the germs feed on them.

New antibiotics will be developed, of course. But so will new armor plating by the germs they are designed to kill.

The most primitive organisms on earth have sat back while their brethren have been killed by the multi-millions, waiting patiently as one or two survived and developed immunity to whatever medicine had been used.

Penicillin was king during World War II, saving countless numbers of human lives while sparing a bacteria or two which went into hiding.

Penicillin had been "discovered" in 1928 by Alexander Fleming, seemingly by accident and intelligent observation, but it did not begin to get used wholesale against bacteria until the late 30's and early 40's. Yet soon after that, in 1946, the doctors discovered a strain of staphylococcus that was immune to penicillin, so in just that short span of time it lost its effectiveness against one of the bacterial killers.

But medicine shrugged its collective shoulder then and dug up another antibiotic ... and staph succumbed once again. *Except for one or two!*

And so it went on decade after decade, new drugs and new mutations. Drugs held a slight lead going into the nineties, and the scourges of the past such as tuberculosis, pneumonia, blood poisoning, syphilis, gonorrhea and other bacterial infections appeared to be vanquished.

But medicine went home a victory or two early.

Every disease-causing bacterium now has strains that are resistant to at least one of medicine's 100-plus antibiotics. Some bacteria resist all but one antibiotic.

Staphylococcus and pneumococcus are nightmare killers. In World War II, 80 percent of the fatalities were from wound infections, not from the wounds themselves. Only one antibiotic still holds these bacteria off. When you develop resistance to that last effective antibacteriacide, you must go beyond man-made drugs. There is no other solution.

Here is a partial listing of antibiotics that are no longer effective against the bacteria they were developed to destroy.

Bacteria	Diseases Caused	Unusable Antibiotics
Enterococcus	blood poisoning surgical infections	erythromycin, penicillin tetracycline, vancomycin, cephalosporins, aminoglycosides.
Haemophilus influenzae	meningitis, ear infections, pneumonia, sinusitis	chloramphenicol, penicillin, tetracycline, trimethoprim/ sulfamethoxazole.
Mycobacterium tuberculosis	tuberculosis	aminoglycosides, ethambutol, isoniazid, pyrazinamide, rifampin.
Neisseria gonorrhoea	gonorrhea	penicillin, spectinomycin, tetracycline.
Plasmodium falciparum	malaria	chloroquine.
Shigella dysenteriae	severe diarrhea	ampicillin, chloramphenicol, tetracycline, trimethoprim/ sulfamethoxazole.
Staphylococcus aureus	blood poisoning pneumonia, surgical infections	all but vancomycin.
Streptococcus pneumoniae	meningitis pneumonia	aminoglycosides, chloram-phemicol, erythromycin, cephalosporins, penicillin, tetracycline, trimethoprim/ sulfamethoxazole.

Staphylo-coccus and pneumo-coccus are nightmare killers. In World War II, 80 percent of the fatalities were from wound infections, not from the wounds themselves.

Scary?

Drug-resistant tuberculosis accounts for one in seven new cases.

Several resistant strains of pneumococcus (children's ear infections, meningitis) appeared in South Africa in the 1970's, spread to Europe and are now showing up in the United States.

In January 1994, the Centers for Disease Control (CDC) reported resistant pneumococcus in Kentucky and Memphis.

In January 1992, doctors reported over 13,000 patients had died of bacterial infections that resisted every antibiotic fired at them. (It wasn't that the bugs resisted every antibiotic, but by the time they went through the list to find an effective one, the patient's immune system had been so compromised that the body was poisoned beyond repair.)

And what about the flesh-eating bacteria? How long will it be before they ride roughshod over the last defending antibiotics?

It should not have come as a surprise that bacteria could follow a "survival of the fittest" route since one bacterium, as we said, can leave almost 17 million offspring in 24 hours.

But there's even more frightening news that renders medical antibiotics more and more useless!

The mutant germs share their resistance gene with their friends and even with unrelated companions.

In these exchanges, E. Coli — a common bacteria found in the human intestines — shares resistance to tetracycline with cholera bacteria. This constitutes a "fast forward" spread of resistance.

What has compounded this medical disaster?

It is you, and every other patient who has demanded antibiotic treatment for situations that could have responded more readily and safely to natural elements. Doctors have given out antibiotics as though they were aspirin, for colds, sore throats, upset stomachs, and even fingernail infections.

It should not have come as a surprise that bacteria could follow a "survival of the fittest" route since one bacterium can leave almost 17 million offspring in 24 hours.

Every dose of antibiotics they prescribed made it easier for resistance to spread because it taught the germs how to overcome these man-made poisons.

And, it is the doctors, who found it "easier" to prescribe antibiotics without investigating the seriousness of the situation, who have also compounded this medical disaster.

Plus the American farmers, who dose their animals with 30 times the amount of penicillin and tetracycline than is given to humans. It was and is economical to treat and prevent disease in animals with antibiotics, and there is the additional bonus that the animals grow faster and plumper with each ounce of antibiotics they are fed.

Because of this, however, drug-resistant microbes emerge in animals the same way they do in you and I and these superbugs can then spread from animals to people! Upwards of 5.1 million people every year get sick from microbes found in meat and poultry.

In the widely hailed British documentary, *The Overworked Miracle*, an American scientist, Dr. Sidney Ross, Chief of Microbiology at the Children's Hospital in Washington, D.C., predicted that this overuse of antibiotics all over the world has actually resulted in more deadly diseases. In Dr. Ross's words, "I think we will be looking back, fifty years hence, at this as being somewhat of a golden era . . . , we may be reverting to the Middle Ages, as far as antibiotic therapy goes!"

It gets worser and worser!

Your children are even more grievously threatened. Their milk, called the world's most perfect food, is *allowed* to contain a concentration of 80 different antibiotics that have been used on dairy cows to prevent udder infection.

Your FDA has set limits on the amounts of antibiotics milk can contain but with every glassful you're getting a minute dose of whatever the cows have been treated with. And now that the FDA has approved bovine growth hormone (BGH) to increase milk production, you'll have to be

Superbugs can spread from animals to people! Upwards of 5.1 million people every year get sick from microbes found in meat and poultry.

> *It's up to you to decide whether you live or die. More than ever, your lifestyle, your diet, your exercise program and your supplement routine will determine how long and how well you'll live.*

careful of more antibiotic contamination because the gene-spliced hormone causes more udder infections.

Are you sufficiently frightened or would you like to learn more about this cataclysmic situation?

Calgene, a biotech company, is considering the preparation of a tomato that will stay fresh longer.

How?

By adding a gene which conveys resistance to the antibiotic kanmycin. If you eat the tomato, chances are the bugs in residence in your stomach will adopt the resistance it brings with it.

In the 1950's, blood poisoning (Staphylococcus aureus) killed up to 80 percent of those it infected. Antibiotics reduced that mortality to less than 5 percent. But now only one antibiotic will kill this persistent microbe. When will this last antibiotic, vancomycin, be overcome and blood poisoning run rampant?

Drug companies are not standing still. New antibiotics are still being discovered. Squalamine from the dogfish shark and Maigainins from the African clawed frog are two recent examples. However, a better strategy might be to abandon antibiotics altogether in favor of different drugs — or even better, improve our own bacteria-fighting abilities.

We must return to the antiseptic routines discovered by Lister to avoid the spread of bacteria. We must use natural antibiotics, such as garlic and echinacea, in place of the easy, now-impotent antibiotic route.

Drug-resistant bacteria don't threaten all of us equally. A healthy immune system can handle most bacterial invaders regardless of their resistance to drugs.

So, once again it's up to you to decide whether you live or die. More than ever, your lifestyle, your diet, your exercise program and your supplement routine will determine how long and how well you'll live. It's up to you to make sure these anti-germotics will now take over and see to it that antibiotics are no longer needed.

Chapter 2

Self Or Not-Self

THE MANDATE OF YOUR IMMUNE SYSTEM, and its essential job, is to distinguish self from not-self, to recognize and take appropriate action against any material that ought not to be in your body, including abnormal and damaged components. It conducts a constant "search and destroy" mission against disease germs in cells infected with germs and viruses. It also recognizes and destroys tumor cells.

Like the nervous system, the immune system is capable of learning. It analyzes its experiences, remembers them, and passes the information on to future generations of cells.

But where is this system and what is it composed of? Until recent years it was not even recognized as a functional part of your body. Even today, surgeons are removing and destroying countless tonsils, adenoids, appendixes and thymus glands under the mistaken impression that these structures are useless, not worth the space they occupied.

But where did *they* get their training?

Your immune system is spread out in your body. It's made up of all those "useless organs," plus your spleen, your bone marrow, the lymph nodes throughout your body and the patches of *lymphoid tissue* found in your intestinal tract.

Whenever your immune system deals successfully with an infection, it emerges from the experience stronger and better able to confront similar threats in the future. Your immune competence develops in combat.

Surgeons are removing and destroying countless tonsils, adenoids, appendixes and thymus glands under the mistaken impression that these structures are useless. . .

A vicious cycle is set up which might be broken by proper nutrition and mega-supplemen-tation.

How does your immune system conduct its guard duties? It's in action from the moment you're born until the day you die, initially supported by antibodies from your mother's milk. White blood cells are the mobile cells which gobble up invaders. B-cells are found in the lymph nodes and the spleen. They produce antibodies which coat invaders and destroy them. The liver and lymph glands strain and detoxify blood and tissue juices. Your thymus gland produces hormones which regulate your immune system and turn your white cells into an active, fighting army.

When an invader is discovered in your body, it is inspected and "photographed," labeled an antigen and put in the lineup. If it is considered to be a new antigen, a specific antibody has to be designed to fit its configurations, like a key made to fit a particular lock. This procedure takes about a week and then the white blood cells are released to search out and destroy the antigen. When the white blood cells locate the invading antigen, they latch on to it and destroy it.

The problem with the AIDS virus is that it carries its own "locksmith" with it, constantly changing locks so that the existing keys don't fit. As long as the virus keeps changing identities, the immune system cannot get a fix and destroy it.

AIDS takes hold more easily in a person whose immune system is already weakened. Then the infection further weakens the system which allows parasites to invade the intestines, causing improper absorption of key nutrients which further weakens the immune response. A vicious cycle is set up which might be broken by proper nutrition and mega-supplementation.

In Africa and Haiti, AIDS is rampant among the nutritionally malnourished and, in America, AIDS victims are usually nutritionally depleted from the use of drugs and the lack of nutritionally-dense foods.

Most humans harbor a fungus called Candida albicans and a parasite called Pneumocystis carinii (PC). A healthy immune system keeps these potential pests in check but if your immune system is compromised these pests can become deadly. In AIDS patients they frequently grow out of bounds and PC is often fatal. A type of cancer called Kaposi's syndrome is common among malnourished African children and was prevalent among Europeans during World War II when food was difficult to obtain. That cancer is frequently seen in AIDS victims, usually young and middle-aged people who are dying so suddenly because their immune systems are compromised and antibiotics have made them so weak they can't even put up a fight. Antibiotics push aside your immune system and kill invading germs all by themselves. Therefore, every time you have another infection, they make your immune system weaker and weaker. To the point that, after five or six antibiotic-treated injections, you've become an immune cripple. You're wide open for even an ordinary attack.

But anti-germotics make your immune system so invulnerable that it slaughters those invading germs solely by itself. Each time your reborn immune system destroys another infection, it grows in strength. It's like playing a sport: the more you practice, the better you are. The power of these anti-germotics has been proven hundreds of times already! There is no longer any question that they work miracles, even where antibiotics miserably fail.

Other nutritional factors also contribute to a weakened immune system. The 20 to 40 year olds who are inflicted with AIDS grew up in an era of junk foods and a relative absence of breast-feeding. This is unfortunate because mother's milk contains a substance called colostrum that is present during the first two to three days of nursing. Besides conferring immunity on the newborn (like a vaccination), it is also a stimulant to the baby's immune system which can last a lifetime.

Anything which damages your general health will have a negative effect on your immune system.

Anti-germotics make your immune system so invulnerable that it slaughters those invading germs solely by itself.

These can all have a negative effect on your immune system.

The following items can all have a negative effect on your total system as well as your immune system:

- Nutritional deficiencies
- Exposure to toxins
- Pollutants
- Infections
- Smoking
- Overuse of alcohol
- Junk food diet
- Exposure to heavy metals like cadmium and mercury

Often the effect of such factors is cumulative and one assault on your body will even magnify the effect of another. Clearly, the first thing you can do to save your immune response is to avoid the harmful ingredient or atmosphere.

Chapter 3

Improving The Immune Response — Vitamins, Minerals and Accessory Nutrients

W HAT ELEMENTS OF NUTRITION have been recommended to strengthen your immune system? There is a forest of suggestions so it's best to identify the trees first and then, later on in this book, talk about the leaves, branches and flowers which can contribute their strengths to strengthen your defense against any invaders.

Vitamin C

Vitamin C is chief among nutrients suggested for strengthening your immune system. Not only is it essential for building your general health, but in the largest doses used (and those doses range up to many grams of vitamin C daily) it will not depress your immune system. Why is this aspect important? It points out one of the overlooked elements which negatively affects your ability to conquer common problems. When you have a cold you take your temperature and, if the fever is in the neighborhood of 100 degrees, you'll probably take two aspirin tablets.

Why?

Because that's what you have been taught to do.

Vitamin C is chief among nutrients suggested for strengthening your immune system.

In volunteers infected with rhinovirus, it was found that aspirin and acetaminophen were associated with suppression of the patient's immune system and therefore increased nasal symptoms and signs.

Certainly, if your temperature rises to a threatening level, you have to take any means to lower it before it can do damage to your body. However, temperature is one of your body's strongest defenses against viral invaders. Viruses reproduce at your body's normal temperature. They prefer the cooler atmosphere. Your body may therefore be smarter than you are. It recognizes that heat can burn up the virus's activity and it begins to turn up the furnace. But you lower the thermostat instead and interfere with the cremation process.

Chinese physicians do not interfere with the immune response. They permit your fever to rise (within reason) and your nose to run.

But there's another reason to avoid taking aspirin or other analgesic products. They can suppress the immune response.

Viruses and Over-The-Counter Drugs

In a double-blind, placebo-controlled trial of over-the-counter analgesic/antipyretic medications (aspirin, acetaminophen, ibuprofen) or placebo in 56 volunteers infected with rhinovirus, it was found that aspirin and acetaminophen were associated with *suppression* of the patient's immune system and therefore *increased* nasal symptoms and signs. There was no difference in viral shedding among the 4 groups, but there was a trend towards longer duration of virus shedding seen in the aspirin and acetaminophen groups.

"Adverse Effects of Aspirin, Acetaminophen, and Ibuprofen on Immune Function, Viral Shedding and Clinical Status in Rhinovirus-Infected Volunteers," Graham, Neil M.H., et al, *The J. of Infectious Diseases*, 1990; 162:1277-1282. (Address: Dr. Graham, Dept. of Epid, Johns Hopkins Sch. of Hyg. & Pub. Hlth, 624 N. Broadway, R895, Baltimore, MD 21205, U.S.A.)

So, doses of vitamin C up to 30 grams a day will not suppress the immune reaction in any way, but two aspirins can. Why? Because your body will eliminate any amount of vitamin C that isn't needed! Therefore, there is no risk of vitamin C poisoning. Results of various studies have supported the theory that vitamin C will enhance immune functioning. One benefit is that it supercharges your body's production of its built-in antivirus interferon. It also enhances humoral aspects of immune function including antibody and complement levels. At the same time, it builds blazing new acceleration into your killer white cells, making those bacterial killers patrol your body at rocket speeds on their endless search for invaders.

CLINICAL GUIDE TO THE USE OF VITAMIN C: Clinical Experiences of Frederick R. Klenner, M.D., 1991, Correspondence: Dr. Lendon Smith, 2233 Southwest Market Street, Portland, Oregon, 97201, Life Sciences Press. This collection of Dr. Frederick Klenner's 30 years of experience with truly "megadoses" of vitamin C in treating all types of illness, including life-threatening disease, is invaluable to the practicing clinician and for that matter to the entire medical profession. Dr. Klenner, a country doctor who specialized in chest diseases, practiced in North Carolina from 1940-1970. His use of truly pharmacological doses of vitamin C (ten to hundreds of grams) ranged from treating poisonous snake bites, polio, and serious burns to meningitis. From his amazing experiences (and those of practitioners today) showing that killer white cells supercharged with megadoses of vitamin C will protect you against any of these invaders mentioned, one can't help but think how ridiculous the discussions sometimes are about the toxicity of vitamin C at milligram dosages, and how important and revealing studies would be using tens to hundreds of grams of vitamin C for acute illness.

Vitamin A

Researchers have studied the relationship between the consumption of vitamin A and the incidence of cancer. These studies have shown that

Vitamin C builds blazing new acceleration into your killer white cells, making those bacterial killers patrol your body at rocket speeds on their endless search for invaders.

Vitamin A strengthens and protects the internal linings of your body. If they are weakened, these membranes in your body can no longer block the entry of germs.

vitamin A, in larger than usual amounts, can protect against the development of cancer and that people who consume high levels of this vitamin are less likely to develop cancer and tumors.

It even appears that vitamin A in the form of beta-carotene can protect against chemical carcinogens and that people who ingested the higher levels of this protection either by consuming green and yellow vegetables and fruits or by supplementation, were less likely to suffer from cancer of the stomach, colon, prostate, etc.

Vitamin A strengthens and protects the internal linings of your body. If they are weakened, these membranes in your body can no longer block the entry of germs.

Early in 1992, Italian scientists reported that a combination of vitamin A and vitamins C and E could correct abnormal cells in the rectum that could eventually progress to cancer. They reported their finding in the *Journal of the National Cancer Institute* (JNCI), 84:47-51.

The use of vitamins in synergistic combination, as in a supplement containing the following, is recommended for immune stimulation as well as a protection against abnormal cells within your body:

- vitamin A   10,000 I.U.
- vitamin C   1,000 mg
- vitamin E   400 I.U.

Beta-carotene slowly reaches more parts of your body and for a longer time; therefore, using both vitamin A and beta-carotene is strongly recommended. Where vitamin A did not significantly reduce the risk of lung cancer, supplements of beta-carotene did.

Beta-carotene also decreases the damage that viruses can do the thymus gland, thereby improving the immune response provided by this important gland. Cytokines are powerful substances manufactured in your body to boost immunity and fight cancer cells. Interferon, interleukin and tumor necrosis factor (TNF) as well as other immune boosters are more active and more in evidence when your body has adequate amounts of beta-carotene.

Unlike vitamin A, beta-carotene can be taken in large amounts without any appreciable harm besides turning your palms and soles orange.

You've Read About Beta-Carotene — But Have You Heard About Its Cousin Alpha-Carotene?

Where does the color of your foods come from?

The color and the health benefits come from about 500 phytochemicals called carotenoids. (Phytochemistry is the chemistry of plants.) The most publicized of them has been beta-carotene with its wonderful health-protecting power of preventing and, in some cases, reversing cancer!

Can we do even better?

How about another carotenoid, perhaps ten times as protective of your body. It's called alpha-carotene. The discovery of this phytochemical was done by Michiaki Murakoshi et al., at the Kyota Prefectual University, Japan. He reported that alpha-carotene suppressed the growth of several types of malignant tumors, including pancreatic cancer and gastric cancer. This was reported in the *Journal of the National Cancer Institute* (Nov. 1, 1989; 81:1649-52). Alpha-carotene began working against cancer cells after just 48 hours and many of those former-cancer cells reversed and began normal activity again. The higher the dose, the greater the benefits.

In follow-up studies it was also found that it was more effective than beta-carotene against liver, lung, and skin cancers. Alpha-carotene, when not immediately needed, is stored in your liver. Perhaps it is also protective of that very important organ while it sits and waits for something nasty to show up.

And still more about phytochemicals like caretenoids. Although we've discovered beta-carotene and alpha-carotene, and have begun to understand their power, there's gamma-carotene on the horizon.

Alpha-carotene suppressed the growth of several types of malignant tumors, including pancreatic cancer and gastric cancer.

Wouldn't it be wonderful if anti-germotics like these took over and antibiotics were no longer needed?

Wouldn't it be wonderful if anti-germotics like these took over and antibiotics were no longer needed?

Alpha-carotene is now available at health food stores. Follow label directions.

While you're in the store, look for a new rival to vitamin E. Vitamin E is a wonderful antioxidant and should be a part of every supplement program, up to 800 I.U. daily, but a new phytochemical derived from, of all things, palm oil, has 100 times the biological antibiotic and anti-microbe power of vitamin E.

And in *Archives of Biochemistry and Biophysics* (Nov. 1, 1989; 532-8) it was first reported that a substance called Lycopene was one of the best dietary antioxidants. (Lycopene is what gives tomatoes and watermelons, for example, their red color.) However, the research wasn't followed up at that time. But when your mother said to eat a lot of color foods, she really knew what she was talking about.

B-Complex Vitamins

The B-Complex vitamins are very important for the general maintenance of your health. They enhance immune function, restore the nutritional status of cancer patients and enhance the effect, while diminishing the side effects, of chemotherapy.

According to researchers at Loma Linda University in Riverside, CA., vitamin B^6 bolsters your immune system, whether obtained from the diet or by supplementation, while a deficiency of B^6 interferes with the formation of DNA and cuts down on the formation of disease-fighting antibodies. Since all the B-Complex vitamins contribute to the immune response, most nutritionists recommend taking all of the B-Complex rather than concentrating on just one or two. A B-50 formula containing 50 mg of the family (50 mcg of B^{12} and 400 mcg of folic acid) taken once in the morning and once at night can be a strong support for your immunity.

Folic Acid

Folic acid, a B vitamin, may be one of the key ingredients in fruits and vegetables that prevents colon cancer, theorize researchers at the Harvard-Medical and Public Health Schools.

Folic acid appears to help the process that turns cancer genes off, according to the researchers, led by Edward Giovannucci of the Harvard Medical School. Alcohol intake, they added, blocks folic acid's action, and may promote cancer.

"This translates into even stronger evidence that we should encourage people to eat as much fruits and vegetables as they can," said Gladys Block, a professor at the University of California, Berkeley, School of Public Health. Government farm policies should be set to enable people to eat more fruits and vegetables, added Dr. Block, who wrote an editorial accompanying the Harvard study, both published in an issue of the *Journal of the National Cancer Institute*.

Process Battles Cancer Genes

The Harvard researchers hypothesize that folic acid helps transfer a compound, called methyl, from molecules commonly found in the body to other molecules that turn off cancer genes. When the process, called methylation, doesn't work as is supposed when alcohol is introduced, cancer genes produce proteins that may cause the cells to proliferate, Dr. Giovannucci said.

The researchers studied 15,984 women between 1980 and 1990, and 9,490 men between 1986 and 1990, who had tests to detect colorectal adenomas, benign tumors that can lead to cancer. Tumors were diagnosed and studied in 564 women and 331 men. The data were drawn from two large epidemiological studies, the Nurses' Health Study and the Health Professionals Follow-Up Study, which studied a broad range of health issues.

Folic acid, a B vitamin, may be one of the key ingredients in fruits and vegetables that prevents colon cancer.

It is recommended that all women of childbearing age take folic acid to prevent birth defects that include paralysis and death.

Analyzing information obtained from questionnaires on the patients' diets during a one-year period, the researchers found that a high intake of folic acid, from fresh fruits and vegetables and vitamin supplements, was associated with a lower risk of developing the tumors. In addition, people who had the equivalent of two alcoholic drinks a day were at an 85 percent higher risk of developing the tumors than nondrinkers.

Folic Acid to Prevent Birth Defects

The United States Public Health Service has recommended that all women of childbearing age should take extra folic acid to prevent neural tube defects that affect 1 to 2 of every 1,000 babies born each year. The effects of these birth defects include paralysis and death.

Researchers on birth defects and nutrition said that if the advice was followed the incidence of neural tube defects like spina bifida and anencephaly should fall to between a quarter and a half of the current figure of 2,300 cases a year.

The recommendation was to take 0.4 milligrams of folic acid a day. Women on average consume just half that amount, said Dr. Irwin Rosenberg, a professor of medicine and nutrition at Tufts University in Boston.

Dr. Steven Laubacher, the executive director of the Spina Bifida Association of America, said, "At our organization, we try to discipline ourselves to be reserved. But this points in the direction of a major, major breakthrough."

Dr. Rosenberg said, "I think this is going to be precedent-setting in respect to the whole business of health claims, supplements and fortification. Let's hope it comes out right."

Neural tube defects include anencephaly, in which most of the brain is missing, and spina bifida, in which a piece of the spinal cord protrudes from the spinal column, causing paralysis of parts of the lower body. Spina bifida also may be accompanied by hydrocephaly, in which fluid fails to drain properly from the skull, a condition that can result in mental retar-dation.

A Study Tips The Scales

Although many researchers had long suspected that folic acid was linked to neural tube defects, the new consensus that folic acid supplements can prevent many of these birth defects was speeded-up by new results from a Hungarian study. These data, on top of a growing pool of other results, were finally enough for some wavering researchers, said Dr. James Mills, the chief of pediatric epidemiology at the National Institute of Child Health and Human Development in Bethesda, Maryland.

A randomized controlled study of women who had not had a previous child with a neural tube defect was completed last spring. It showed that low doses of folic acid can prevent neural tube defects in these women. "It was very persuasive," Dr. Mills said. "It tipped the scales."

The new advice was formulated by scientists who met at the Centers for Disease Control, said Dr. Godfrey Oakley, who directs research on birth defects at the disease centers in Atlanta.

But the advice raises a thorny question. How are women supposed to get this folic acid? It is not enough to tell them to take the vitamin after they are pregnant because the birth defects occur when the fetus's spinal column is fusing, at about two weeks after the first missed menstrual period. Many women do not even know they are pregnant at that time, which is why they are advised to consume the folic acid if they are even capable of becoming pregnant. Vegetables like spinach and broccoli are especially rich in folic acid. But a lot of vegetables must be eaten to ingest 0.4 milligrams of folic acid a day, which is about twice the amount recommended by the National Academy of Sciences for men and women aged 15 to 30. Women would have to eat about one and a half cups of boiled spinach to get the recommended amount of folic acid, and many people just do not eat green vegetables in such doses.

It is not enough to tell women to take the vitamin after they are pregnant because the birth defects occur when the fetus's spinal column is fusing, at about two weeks after the first missed menstrual period.

Another possibility is to fortify foods, in much the same way that vitamin D is added to milk to prevent rickets and iodine is added to salt to prevent goiters. The Spina Bifida Association and leading researchers, including Dr. Aubrey Milunsky of Boston University, urge this course. But Dr. David A. Kessler, the Commissioner of the Food and Drug Administration, says he is undecided.

"That's an issue we need to confront as an agency," Dr. Kessler said. He said he was hesitant to take such a course because folic acid supplements can mask pernicious anemia, a disorder mainly of older people. "By doing good, we don't want to do harm," he said. He added that he was concerned about evaluating health claims by food manufacturers.

Methionine, An Amino Acid, May Also Help

An amino acid, methionine, may also provide the same protection as folic acid, the researchers found. Methionine is found in fish and chicken.

The findings add to a growing body of evidence that several factors may be at work in the prevention of colon cancer, said Dr. Gladys Block of the UC Berkeley School of Public Health in the *Journal of The National Cancer Institute*. Other vitamins and nutrients, such as vitamins C and E and carotenoids, also appear to work against cancer, she added. The evidence on fiber is mixed, in part because many studies assumed the benefit of fruit intake was from the fiber, she said. A second study in the Journal confirms that diets high in saturated fats and low in carbohydrates, fruits and vegetables may increase cancer risk.

Diets high in saturated fats and low in carbohydrates, fruits and vegetables may increase cancer risk.

Although some health experts recommend against taking vitamin supplements in place of fruits and vegetables, Dr. Block advocates supplements and fortifying prepared foods because most people don't eat balanced diets. "Nutritionists would say they ought to eat the whole fresh fruit, and I agree," she said, "but they're not."

Zinc

Zinc acts in synergy with vitamin A in preventing thymus and lymph atrophy from stress, injury, surgery, aging, radiation and infection. A zinc deficiency can cause a severe depression of antibody production, and causes a depletion of both T and B lymphocyte populations. A zinc deficiency impairs PGE-1 synthesis from GLA.

Zinc is recognized as an element which strengthens the immune system. It takes part in over 200 chemical reactions in your body and has been shown to shorten the duration of a cold or even short-circuit it entirely.

But how much zinc and what kind?

Zinc lozenges, taken every two hours at the first sign of a cold, can shortstop the cold and eliminate the need for any thought of antibiotic therapy. Doctors frequently prescribe such therapy to "prevent" a possible secondary infection. That concept has led to the problem of bacterial tolerance to antibiotics.

Godrey, J.C., Sloane, B.C. et al: Zinc gluconate and the common cold: a controlled clinical study. *J Internal Med Res* 20:234-246,1992.

In a randomized, placebo-controlled, double-blind study, zinc gluconate/glycine lozenges were examined for their effectiveness in relieving symptoms of the common cold. All subjects voluntarily reported to the Dartmouth College Health Service with at least 2/9 predetermined cold symptoms, and were instructed to self-administer lozenges every two hours up to eight times daily until symptoms abated. In the group receiving zinc lozenges (n=35), as well as in the group receiving a zinc-free placebo (n=38), median age was 20-21 years, and males outnumbered females by a significant margin. At 7 days following symptom onset, self-reported diary data showed 15 total symptoms remaining in the group which had received zinc supplements, as compared with 45 total symptoms in the group which had received a zinc-free placebo. Average disappearance of all symptoms occurred for experimental subjects at 4.9 days, versus 6.1

Zinc lozenges, taken every two hours at the first sign of a cold, can shortstop the cold and eliminate the need for antibiotics.

The critical role of zinc in immune cell function has gained widespread attention in nutritional research.

days for controls. Subjects taking zinc-gluconate/glycine lozenges averaged 8 lozenges/day, each containing 23.7 mg/zinc for a total of 189.6 mg/day total intake.

Researchers selected a zinc gluconate/glycine delivery formula based on its high rate of release of zinc ions in the mouth (90-93 percent). They hypothesized that disappointing results from previous zinc gluconate studies involved the deactivation of zinc ions through chelation with other lozenge components, including citric acid, tartaric acid, and mannital/sorbitol.

Thanks largely to the work of RK Chandra and colleagues at the Johns Hopkins School of Hygiene and Public Health, the critical role of zinc in immune cell function has gained widespread attention in nutritional research. The ability of zinc to modify activity of lymphocytes, neutrophils, and natural killer cells has been well documented.

So, take it every two hours at the first sign of a cold and see it stop that cold dead in its tracks, eliminating any need for antibiotics.

Glutathione

Glutathione is one of the most important antioxidant defense mechanisms in the body. Sufficient levels of glutathione are responsible for protecting cells from the damaging effects of certain free radicals. Glutathione and vitamin C have a very close relationship in the body. Vitamin C maintains glutathione in a state that makes it an optimal antioxidant. As vitamin C levels decrease, glutathione ceases to act as an effective defense mechanism. Conversely, glutathione promotes the antioxidant activity of vitamin C. Normal activity of both of these constituents is essential to maintaining cell health and normal immunity.

Johnston, C.S., Meyer, C.G. & Srilakshmi: Vitamin C elevates red blood cell glutathione in healthy adults. *Amer J Clin Nutr* 58: 103-5, 1993.

The effect of supplemental ascorbic acid (vitamin C) on red blood cell glutathione levels was examined in 9 healthy adults (18 to 50 years in age).

Subjects consumed a vitamin-C-restricted diet, then received placebo for the first week, 500 mg of ascorbic acid (L-ascorbate) for weeks 2 and 3, 2,000 mg of ascorbic acid for weeks 5 and 6, and placebo for week 6. Average red blood cell (RBC) glutathione rose nearly 50 percent after a single week of the 500 mg period when compared to the first week of placebo.

This is not to suggest that using higher doses of vitamin C at the beginning of a cold or flu may not be useful. Another issue that this study does not address is optimal, daily intake of vitamin C in immunosuppressed individuals (e.g. HIV-infection, cancer). The glutathione system in these individuals is severely taxed and often functioning sub-optimally. Taking the above study design to this population in an attempt to identify optimal daily intake of vitamin C is a logical next step.

Carnitine

We've heard a lot about carnitine as a weight-reduction nutrient since it helps feed fatty acids from your bloodstream into your cell's engine to be burned — like coal — for energy.

It is found in meat but can also be manufactured in your body when there are appreciable amounts of the amino acids lysine and methionine plus B^3, B^6, iron and vitamin C present.

There has been considerable debate over whether or not to consider carnitine a vitamin. A recent review concluded that it is an essential nutrient, especially in infancy, pregnancy, fasting, and breast-feeding, even though technically it can be manufactured in your body. But vitamin or essential nutrient, it can influence the course of cancer. This is due to its influence on the mitochondria (the cell's furnace).

It is known that responses of thymus-mediated white blood cells slow as people age but that white blood cells proliferated when carnitine was present, leaving more cells to roam and locate antigens. In addition, when carnitine was present, it protected white blood cells attacked by free rad-

Glutathione promotes the antioxidant activity of vitamin C. Normal activity of both is essential to cell health and normal immunity.

icals, so, even though most people's immune systems fall apart as they age, yours won't if carnitine is present.

L-Carnitine is available in health food stores, by itself or in combination with other nutrients.

Quercitin

Quercitin is a flavonoid derived from the common horse chestnut and other common fruits and vegetables. The Japanese have discovered that it markedly inhibited the growth of human cancer cells. (Yoshida, M. et al. *Febs. Lett.* 1990; 260: 10-3)

Quercitin inhibits the infectivity of the herpes virus according to an article in the *Journal of Allergy and Clinical Immunology* (82;60:104). In other words, it pulls the fangs out of the herpes virus, whether it attacks your mouth, lips or elsewhere — stops its spread cold. The killer virus now passes through your body like water. Harmless water. It's still alive, it just can't reach out and infect you.

Quercitin also stabilizes the walls of cells that contain histamine which can cause the allergic reactions to antigens, thus blocking allergic reactions — in seconds.

To get enough of this one anti-germotic, quercitin, you would have to eat so much of the foods that contain it — grapefruits (the white portion directly below the skin), onions, apples, broccoli and summer squash — that you would spend half your day on the toilet. Since it is so difficult to digest and to obtain in the quantities that prove helpful, doesn't it make sense to take 3 tiny pills as supplements instead? The recommended dosage for maintenance, or as a preventive measure, is a mixture of bioflavanoids, 200 to 500 mg daily, or 50 to 150 mg of quercitin. Vitamin C should be part of this formula since it multiplies the beneficial effects.

Quercitin pulls the fangs out of the herpes virus, whether it attacks your mouth, lips or elsewhere— stops its spread cold. The killer virus now passes through your body like water. It's still alive, it just can't reach out and infect you.

A combination of quercitin and the pineapple-derived digestant bromelain make the quercitin easier to assimilate. This is particularly important for the more mature individual.

One of the other benefits of this bioflavonoid is its ability to slow or halt the oxidation of LDL, the bad cholesterol, (*Biochem Pharmacol* 90;39:1743-59) while it reduces the stickiness of the platelets in your blood, making blood clots so slippery they can't stick to your artery walls.

So quercitin protects your arteries at the same time that it stands guard to ward off cancer cells. It is available in most health food stores.

Vitamin E

This favorite vitamin is a powerful antioxidant which prevents membrane rancidity.

Excess vitamin E increases antibody response to germs up to two to three times the norm (in vitamin E-deficient animals, there is lessened or no antibody response at all).

Vitamin E is involved in T-lymphocyte's stimulation of B cells to make antibodies and increases T-helper cells activity.

Experimental animals given excess vitamin E increase their resistance to infection and exhibit a four-fold increase in survival rates. So, to survive you must take excess vitamin E. Forget doctors' baby doses. Only giant intakes will protect you against super germs.

Animals given excess vitamin E exhibit a four-fold increase in survival rates. Forget doctors' baby doses. Only giant intakes will protect you against super germs.

Gamma Linoleic Acid

Gamma linoleic acid (GLA) is the precursor to PGE-1, the prostaglandin which is a key regulator of T-lymphocyte function. GLA, in theory, can be made in the body from vegetable oil but, in practice, a deficiency in any of the following — vitamins B^3, B^6, C, zinc, magnesium, or vitamin A — can block the process. Also, excess trans-fatty acids from margarine and other hydrogenated oils, a high-fat diet, some viruses, aging, radiation, or diabetes may interfere with its production.

Rather than take chances, supplement your diet with evening primrose oil (two capsules with meals), black currant seed oil or borage oil. If they are not to your liking, pure GLA is available at your health store. Follow label directions.

Magnesium

Magnesium is required for the activation of the alternative pathway of the complement system (blood proteins that help destroy germs). Magnesium is necessary for phagocytes to ingest and kill germs. If there is insufficient magnesium in your body, thymus gland atrophy can occur along with a significant reduction in antibody levels.

Iron

Iron deficiency causes decreased numbers of T and B lymphocytes and reduces the ability of macrophages to kill and digest microbes.

Selenium

Selenium is a powerful antioxidant and key partner/synergist with vitamin E. It is essential for a key enzyme, glutathione peroxidase, which detoxifies hydrogen peroxide that leaks into the tissues.

Selenium stimulates increased antibody response to germ infections as much as 30-fold in some experiments. From just one pill a day, your immune cells have 30 times the infection-fighting power.

Organic Germanium

Germanium (GE-132) increases the activity of gamma interferon, a key body-produced immunostimulant. In human volunteers, GE-132

From just one pill a day, your immune cells have 30 times the infection-fighting power.

increased T and B-cell activity, NK (natural killer) cells, and antibody dependent cellular cytotoxicity, as well as the numbers of antibody-forming cells.

Organic germanium was taken off the market at one point because there were reports that inorganic germanium had been implicated in causing liver problems in some people. However, it is *inorganic* germanium that was the culprit, not the organic kind. So be sure you buy organic germanium.

Coenzyme Q-10

CoQ-10 increases the phagocytic activity of macrophages (very large white blood cells) and has improved survival time in induced infections with various germs and strains of bacteria.

CoQ-10 increases levels of IgG antibodies. It improves cellular energy metabolism — the billions of immune cells require massive amounts of energy for their constant production, surveillance, and germ and cancer cell-killing activities. In other words, it gives your immune cells explosive new energy, feeding billions of them every hour.

CoQ-10 gives your immune cells explosive new energy, feeding billions of them every hour.

L-Cysteine

L-cysteine is a sulfur-containing amino acid that is necessary to the production of glutathione, a major detoxifying chemical used by your liver and lymphocytes to neutralize chemical and germ poisons. It is a powerful detoxifier of alcohol and tobacco smoke, both potent immune suppressers and disease susceptibility factors.

It is a thymus-protecting antioxidant that also protects the phagocytes from free radicals as they patrol your body and destroy germs.

Egg Lecithin

Another valuable booster for the immune system is egg lecithin. At the Weizmann Institute in Israel, when the 7:2:1 form of egg lecithin was administered to over-50 people whose weakened immune systems were ready to collapse, those crippled immune systems first returned to normal, and then continued to strengthen until they were stronger than people dozens of years younger.

The ratio shown is 70 percent neutral lipids, 20 percent phosphatidyl choline and 10 percent phosphatidyl ethanolamine. This product is available in health food stores.

In over-50 people, those crippled immune systems first returned to normal, and then continued to strengthen until they were stronger than people dozens of years younger.

Chapter 4

Immune Defense Force

Y OUR IMMUNE SYSTEM IS HELPLESS without daily reinforcements from natural foods and supplements.

That's why your body grows more vulnerable as you grow older. Not because your immune cells are dying of old age. Far from it! It's because you're starving them to death — for these reinforcements they need every day.

Your immune defense force is a combination of natural body products supported by other natural products from your diet or from supplements.

We can call these cells immune system tigers! They not only eat invading bacteria and viruses, but also molds, chemicals, fungi, pollution and parasites, as detailed below.

- Acid and stomach enzymes are capable of digesting bacteria, molds and parasites.

- Phagocytes are white blood cells capable of ingesting chemical and cellular debris as well as bacteria, viruses and fungi.

- Skin and mucous-lined epithelial cells, which line the nose, mouth, throat, lungs and stomach, provide a physical barrier to keep germs out of your body. Healthy mucous cells secrete enzymes which are capable of dissolving microbes the instant they land on their territory. Exposing viruses to immune forces this strong is like dropping water on a red-hot stove. That's why you don't just get weaker infections than your neighbors! You get no infections at all!

Exposing viruses to immune forces this strong is like dropping water on a red-hot stove. You don't just get weaker infections! You get no infections at all!

☐

They're on their way! Colds that kill and flu that kills, but they'll bounce right off you if you have fortified your immune system.

☐

- Macrophages are special types of phagocytes which are in lymphoid tissue: Lymph nodes, lungs, liver, sinus cells, spleen and bone marrow. They can ingest many types of germs and toxins.

- B-Lymphocytes are cells that transform upon exposure to invading germs into immune factories for various germ-specific antibodies. Antibodies and other complement factors, often called "humoral immunity" are blood-borne proteins made by B-cells that spew out billions of immune guided missiles which are attracted to the specific germs the antibodies have been manufactured to destroy and which blow apart the attacking germs.

- T-helper lymphocytes help direct B-cells to which antibodies to make.

- T-effecter cells help destroy bacteria.

- T-suppresser cells turn off the killer branch of your immune system after it has successfully destroyed the invaders.

If you expose yourself to particularly virulent microorganisms like the one that causes gonorrhea, there's a 99 percent chance that you will come down with the disease. However, if a group of people are exposed to the germs which cause colds and flu, those people with a strong immune system will not be affected.

They're on their way! Colds that kill and flu that kills, but they'll bounce right off you if you have fortified your immune system.

Bacteria and viruses have completely outwitted our man-made poisons, but no bacteria or virus can outwit being eaten like a cheese sandwich!

Now you have this different kind of weapon against these invisible killers: the anti-germotics!

What is an anti-germotic? It is a natural substance, therefore it does not battle bacteria and viruses by trying to poison them (and also poison your body), like antibiotics do. Instead, it builds explosive new power into your body's own killer cells, and allows those natural defenders to tear apart germs the instant they invade your body!

It makes no difference whether you're under attack by bacteria or viruses! These killer cells don't care! The very moment these germs break into your system, these killer cells engulf the invaders. In a split second, they eat them, dissolve them and digest them, then spit them out as gar-bage — then they go on to the next wave of invaders and the next and next.

The bacteria, the viruses never have a chance. They never have a second to divide and reproduce. They are simply ripped to shreds by billions of your own super-powered killing and eating cells.

And the results! They prevent super colds and super flu.

The bacteria, the viruses never have a chance. They are simply ripped to shreds by billions of your own super-powered killing and eating cells.

Chapter 5

Antioxidants

ANTIOXIDANTS SHOW PROMISE IN CANCER THERAPY. Tucson, Ariz.—Two new studies have shown that antioxidants can aid in the regression of some oral and cervical cancers, according to researchers.

In one study of 49 patients with oral leukoplakia, a regimen of 60 mg/day of beta-carotene resulted in regression of lesions in 26 patients over six months, reported Harinder Garewal M.D., Ph.D., assistant director of Cancer Prevention and Control at the Tucson VA Medical Center and the Arizona Cancer Center. The regressions occurred even in patients who kept smoking. Dr. Garewal made his presentation at the American Cancer Society Science Writer's Seminar.

In an another report, Scott Lippman, M.D., of M.D. Anderson Cancer Center reported on 32 patients with advanced cervical cancer who received a combination of oral 13-cisretinoic acid and subcutaneous alpha interferon. Half of his patients had at least a 50 percent regression in the size of very large tumors — up to 20 cm in some cases. Another 27 patients have also completed the regimen and a multinational trial in the U.S., Mexico, Brazil and Argentina is expected to determine the effect on survival of this type of treatment.

"We have actually treated a number of types of cancers in phase II trials over the last years, and we've seen activity in squamous cell carcinomas of the skin and now in the cervix," Dr. Lippman said. "We have not seen

Half of his patients had at least a 50 percent regression in the size of very large tumors.

activity in advanced sqamous cell carcinomas of the head and neck, or of the lung, or in melanoma. So there seems to be something specific about cervical cancer. It's possible the favorable results could be due to the viral etiology of the disease."

Treating premalignant lesions or cancer with antioxidants is a logical approach, said Margaret Hanausek, Ph.D., assistant biochemist and assistant professor of carcinogenesis at M.D. Anderson. "However, I think this has to be done in a very controlled setting where we are not doing more harm than good," because of the potential for toxicity, she said. As for chemoprevention, Dr. Hanausek said she believes that the best approach is a good diet.

Herbal Antioxidants

Rediscovering what the ancients knew — plants can be powerful medicine.

When people today hear the word "antioxidants," they think of vitamins like A, C, and E. People, however, have taken antioxidants as medicines for thousands of years, in the form of plants. Nearly 2,000 years ago, Pliny the Elder, the Roman naturalist, wrote about medicinal uses of milk thistle. Today's research reveals that milk thistle is a strong antioxidant. Another plant that scientists now know acts as an antioxidant — ginkgo — was likely used as a medicine for even longer. Ginkgo, the world's oldest tree species, is estimated to be 200 million years old. Traces of its medicinal use date back at least several thousand years. Milk thistle and ginkgo are two herbal antioxidants that modern scientists have studied the most, but as research continues, we are likely to learn of many others.

Many people who take antioxidant vitamins are aware that these nutrients "fight" chemically reactive free radicals in the body. Free radicals are highly reactive atoms on molecules that can damage cells and cause genetic mutation. Scientists today attribute many diseases, as well as aging of the

Plants can be powerful medicine. Herbal antioxidants "fight" chemically reactive free radicals in the body.

Antioxidants offer protection against oxygen-free radicals circulating in the body that are related to infections, heart and artery complications, arthritis and a depressed immune system.

body, to the damage caused by free radicals. They also suspect that modern conditions such as high-fat diets and our increasing exposure to chemical pollutants have increased the health threats posed by free radicals.

Milk thistle could become a potent antidote to that threat, particularly since it has proved to act effectively in the liver, where poisonous chemicals are detoxified. Milk thistle (Silybum marianum) is a biennial plant native to the Mediterranean region and southwest Europe and has been cultivated for centuries as a food and as a medicinal and ornamental plant. The use of milk thistle gradually spread to northern Europe — records show that the British ate its peeled, boiled stalks and tiny artichoke-like flower receptacles. They also used the seed as a coffee substitute. Today, milk thistle grows wild in the eastern United States and in California.

Antioxidants, Not Antibiotics

Because of the complications of heart disease, cancer, angina and other health conditions, government agencies have been encouraging Americans to consume more fruits and vegetables each day since they are rich sources of such antioxidants as vitamin A, beta-carotene, vitamin C, vitamin E and so forth. Unfortunately, almost 72 percent of the adult population do not eat fruits and vegetables rich in vitamin C daily, and almost 80 percent of Americans do not consume foods rich in vitamin A each day. Further, almost 47 percent of women between the ages of 19 and 50 have a daily intake of vitamin E that is less than 70 percent of the Recommended Dietary Allowance.

Antioxidants are important to human health because they offer protection against oxygen-free radicals circulating in the body that are related to infections, heart and artery complications, arthritis and a depressed immune system. In a word, an antioxidant prevents a reaction between various food constituents and oxygen. A typical reaction is when oxygen reacts with a cut apple so that it turns brown.

Although free radicals are a byproduct of metabolism, especially when they react with fat molecules, they can also be generated by such environmental factors as excessive sunlight, molds, dust, noise, air and water pollution, among others.

"Mounting scientific evidence supports the hypothesis that diet may play a broader role in heart disease than simply affecting blood cholesterol levels," according to Charles H. Hennekens, M.D., Dr.P.H. in *VNIS Backgrounder*. "Furthermore, heart disease risk reduction through diet modification has become more widely accepted, with a new focus on increased intakes of protective factors rather than decreased intakes of causative and contributory agents. Study of the roles of antioxidant vitamins — vitamin C, vitamin E and beta-carotene — in protecting against heart disease is a rapidly growing area of research."

Diet may play a broader role in heart disease than simply affecting blood cholesterol levels.

Chapter 6

Phytochemicals

PHYTOCHEMICALS (chemicals found naturally in foods) extend beyond the known vitamins and minerals. Research has uncovered dozens of totally new health-protecting substances and these anti-germotics must be part of your daily diet. If you object to the taste of the food or the smell and wouldn't make it part of your table, however, you can find most of the phytochemicals listed in tablets at your local health food store.

Research has uncovered dozens of totally new health-protecting substances and these anti-germotics must be part of your daily diet.

Phytochemicals In Foods

Although no food or food combination has yet been clinically proven to prevent or retard disease in people, research strongly suggests that many components have specific biological reactions that may prove helpful. Scientists suspect compounds would have to be extracted and given in larger doses than those found naturally.

Component	Possible disease-fighting properties	Food sources
ALLYLIC SULFIDES	May protect against carcinogens by stimulating production of a detoxificaion enzyme, glutathione-S-transferase.	Garlic and onions.
CAROTENOIDS (vitamin A precursors)	Antioxidants and cell differentiation agents (cancer cells are non-differentiated).	Parsley, carrots, winter squash, sweet potoes, yams, apricots, spinach, kale, turnip greens, citrus fruit.
CATECHINS (tannins)	Antioxidants, linked to lower rates of gastro-intestinal cancer; mechanisms not understood.	Green tea, berries.

Component	Possible disease-fighting properties	Food sources
FLAVONOIDS	Block receptor sites for certain hormones that promote cancers.	Most fruits and vegetables, including parsley, carrots, citrus fruits, broccoli, cabbage, cucumbers, squash, yams, tomatoes, eggplant, peppers, soy products, berries.
GENISTEIN	In test tubes, blocks anglogenesis, the growth of new blood vessels essential for some tumors to grow and spread, and deters proliferation of cancer cells.	Found in urine of people with diets rich in soy-beans and, to a lesser extent, cabbage-family vegetables.
FIBER	Dilutes carcinogenic compounds in colon and speeds them through digestive system; discourages growth of harmful bacteria while bolstering healthful ones; may encourage production of healthier form of estrogen.	Whole grains and many vegetables.
INDOLES	Induce protective enzymes.	Cabbage, Brussels sprouts, kale.
ISOTHIO-CYANATES	Induce protective enzymes.	Mustard, horseradish, radishes.
LIMONOIDS	Induce protective enzymes.	Citrus fruits.
LINOLENIC ACID	Regulates prostaglandin production.	Many leafy vegetables and seeds, especially flaxseed.
LYCOPENE	Antioxidant.	Tomatoes, red grapefruit.
MONO-TERPENES	Some antioxidant properties; inhibit cholesterol production in tumors; aid protective enzyme activity.	Parsley, carrots, broccoli, cabbage, tomatoes, eggplant, peppers, mint, basil, citrus.
PHENOLIC ACIDS (tannins)	Some antioxidant properties; inhibit formation of nitrosamine, a harmful carcinogen, and affect enzyme activity.	Parsley, carrots broccoli, cabbage, tomatoes, eggplant, peppers, citrus fruits, whole grains, berries.
PLANT STEROLS (vitamin D precursors)	Differentiation agents.	Broccoli, cabbage, cucumbers, squash, yams, tomatoes, egg-plant, peppers, soy products, whole grains.
VITAMIN C	Antioxidant; inhibits creation of nitrosamine in the stomach.	Citrus fruits, tomatoes, green leafy vegetables, potatoes.
VITAMIN E	Antioxidant.	Wheat germ, oatmeal, peanuts, nuts, brown rice.

Dilutes carcinogenic compounds in colon and speeds them through the digestive system.

From **The Medical Tribune**

Vitamin Supplements May Help
Delay Onset of AIDS

With the FDA and the AMA in an avoidance and denial mode when it comes to supplemental nutrition, this headline appears to show a recognition of what the "health nuts" have been talking about for so long.

A healthy diet and supplemental vitamins may delay the onset of AIDS in HIV-positive men, according to research done at the University of California, Berkeley.

"Roughly one-third less of the people who took multivitamin supplements developed AIDS compared with those who did not," said Barbara Abrams of the School of Public Health.

Although the article did not specify the supplements or amounts, outside of praising iron and vitamin E, a strong multi-vitamin/mineral formula supported by extra A, beta-carotene, C, selenium, E and perhaps alpha-carotene would probably fit the supplement profile. The recommended high-carbohydrate, high-fiber, low-fat diet would handle the food portion, along with low-salt, low-sugar, low-alcohol consumption.

Certainly worth a try!

Roughly one-third less of the people who took multivitamins developed AIDS. Certainly worth a try!

Chapter 7

Mothers Milk . . . Colostrum — Not Just For Babies

MOTHER'S MILK is the original health food!

After three million some odd years, we've discovered one of the most important supplements ever produced by Mother Nature, and babies get it for nothing.

But, it's not just for babies anymore.

It's been discovered that mother's milk offers a wide spectrum of health benefits for adults — from enhanced immunity to improved physical fitness.

This is not license to suckle on the first available breast. There's more to health benefits than that, and it's only the milk that's secreted during the first 24 to 72 hours after giving birth. That antibody-rich substance is called colostrum, and it's nature's way of passing immunity from mother to child.

It may also be a way to achieving lifelong health and fitness.

Your body is constantly being bombarded by millions of disease-causing organisms. If they are able to penetrate your natural shields, the body initiates an immune response in an attempt to ward off the invaders. However, unless your body has been invaded by that particular organism before, it may take several days or even weeks to get a partial or full response. In

It offers a wide spectrum of health benefits for adults — from enhanced immunity to improved physical fitness.

> *These anti-disease immune superchargers and immune tigers cannot be found in as high a concentration in any other natural substance. It's like having Instant Immunity.*

the meantime, disease symptoms appear as a result of cell destruction. If enough destruction is accomplished . . . the victim may die!

The importance of a strong immune system has never been as apparent as now. The AIDS epidemic has brought that to our attention and research is showing that immune deficiencies are also linked to cancer, chronic fatigue symptoms, and a host of other devastating illnesses. In fact, scientists are now beginning to trace these illnesses to immune deficiencies that open the body up, first of all, to infection, and then to the cancer, chronic fatigue and the rest.

What has this to do with colostrum?

Colostrum contains an abundance of nutritional factors necessary to enhance the immune response of a newborn. These anti-disease immune superchargers and immune tigers cannot be found in as high a concentration in any other natural substance. Plus, there is a unique combination of high energy nutrients and other elements necessary for growth. And protective antibodies such as immunoglobulins, growth factors, immunity-regulating peptides and other biological regulators. And still more, a factor that stimulates the assimilation and use of all of the biological factors so that nothing is lost.

Colostrum covers such a large spectrum that it can provide protection not only for the infant but for people of all ages.

It's like having Instant Immunity — exactly as though you had the disease before and conquered it. That protection from the colostrum is why you suffer no symptoms at all!

And don't let them fool you! Cancer can be triggered by an infection, so can chronic fatigue, and so can a host of other devastating illnesses.

Research on colostrum is continuing, since it is so unbelievably powerful that it not only blocks infections but may also treat arthritis, diabetes and other body insults. In non-insulin-dependent diabetes, it increases the body's uptake of blood glucose. Its concentration of insulin-like growth factors may be able to take up where insulin leaves off in transporting glucose and amino acids into cells.

Other concepts under investigation are:

- prevention and treatment of viral infections
- treatment of AIDS-related disease
- healing of tissue and muscle damage
- treatment of diarrhea and digestive disorders
- treatment of allergies

Colostrum has also caught the interest of fitness-minded individuals because of its anabolic and fat-burning properties and its workout-recovery effects.

It appears to contain potent growth-stimulating substances which resemble insulin in activity. They promote protein synthesis and build muscle, but block fat storage, an ideal situation for the athlete and for the dieter. After a hard workout the growth factors increase your body's muscle-growing ability while slowing down catabolism (muscle breakdown), thus, assisting in muscular development.

The insulin-like growth factors in colostrum have a more potent anabolic effect on muscle cells than any other compound known. Perhaps even strong enough to rival the effects of steroids. In addition, colostrum contains a substance that will actually facilitate repair of injured tissue.

Boy! Somebody ought to patent the stuff and put it on prescription.

Luckily, it's available at health food stores. No, they're not kidnapping women and stealing their milk. Thanks to modern technology, the health benefits are in good supply, although there's a lot of calves that may complain. Cow's colostrum is virtually identical to human issue. It is obtained during the first 36 hours postpartum, processed under strict control to get rid of any bacteria, pasteurized, and is then ready for human consumption.

Take about 250 mg daily to enhance your immune system or follow label directions if you're building your body. There are no side effects and no overdose has ever been reported.

And say "thank you" to your mother!

There are no side effects and no overdose has ever been reported.

Chapter 8

Herbs

> □
>
> *The antibacterial properties of garlic have been shown to devastate a variety of bacteria, including streptococcus bacteria, the blood poisoning and surgical infection killer.*
>
> □

PENICILLIN is a sulfur derivative.

Garlic contains a number of sulfur derivatives.

It took less than a decade for bacteria to develop resistant strains to penicillin.

It's been over 5,000 years since garlic has been used as an anti-germotic antibiotic and it's still killing germs and none of them have developed immunity to its killing power!

Garlic contains a number of sulfur compounds, the most biologically active being allicin which is activated when whole fresh garlic is cut or crushed. Allicin is responsible for garlic's odor. But more important, it's what gives garlic its medicinal punch. In an October 1991 study (Weber, N.D. et al. In vitro virucidal effects of Allium sativum (garlic) extract and compounds. *Planta Medica*, 1992; 58:417-423) researchers found that the higher the levels of allicin and other compounds in various garlic preparations, the greater the killing power on such viruses as herpes simplex, parainfluenza (super influenza) and rhinovirus.

Clinical studies of the antibacterial properties of garlic have shown all forms to devastate a variety of bacteria including: streptococcus bacteria, the blood poisoning and surgical infection killer . . . salmonella enteritis, the ruthless food poisoner and cause of weeks-long diarrhea . . . and staphylococcus aureus, the source of the great new plague of pneumonia.

And all these killers are the ones that have proven to be more and more invulnerable to antibiotics.

In one study, a crude extract of garlic was put in a petri dish with other antibiotics and found to disable all strains of bacteria, even more than all antibiotics except chloramphenicol.

If you're laid low with a cold or flu, slice a couple of cloves of garlic and blend with a glass of grapefruit juice and lemon juice. Take this mixture three times a day for ten days as if it were a super-antibiotic, because that's just what it is.

If this is too strong for your liking, take two garlic tablets three times a day for ten days.

So, if garlic is still killing germs and none of them have developed immunity to it, what does this say about the use of natural herbs as the first resort against most super-bacterial and super-viral invasions? That these superbugs can't overwhelm these natural anti-germotics because the anti-germotics are hundreds of times more sophisticated than the out-dated antibiotics.

Herbs are plants or plant parts valued for their medicinal, savory or aromatic qualities. The four great herbal traditions — Egyptian-European, Native American, Indian and Chinese — have each contributed to our health and well-being. It is only in the last century that synthetic chemical compounds have emerged from the laboratory, but even so, about half of all drugs in use today are derived from plants.

In cancer, such conventional agents as vincristine, vinblastine, maytansine, podophyllium and taxol are all derived from plants, some of which were native remedies before being discovered and refined in the laboratory.

These superbugs can't overwhelm these natural anti-germotics! The anti-germotics are hundreds of times more sophisticated than the outdated antibiotics.

Can Animals Teach Us Medicine?

The literature of tropical natural history indicates that many animals, particularly monkeys, pigs, and elephants, use plants as medicines as well

Animals find and eat true medicinal plants. Perhaps we can identify useful medical plants by observing the practices of the animal kingdom.

as food. These animals find and eat true medicinal plants orally, topically, and by buccal administration. Ethiopian baboons at risk of schistosomiasis ingest Balanites fruits, which are rich in the potent antischistosome diosgenin, while those not exposed do not eat them. Chimpanzees massage the leaves of the Aspilia plant between their tongue and cheek before swallowing it. Aspilia, which is an important African traditional medicine, has potent antibiotic and antifungal activity. The active principle probably passes across the buccal mucosa, but is destroyed by gastric acidity. Other animals have been found to use antidiarrheal agents and various psychoactive drugs.

Many of the effective medicines used by humans were originally derived from plants. So far, only one percent of the world's plants have been investigated for possible medical applications. Perhaps we can identify useful medical plants by observing the practices of the animal kingdom. As we continue to degrade the rain forests, many of these plants face extinction. (The American Botanical Council.)

Herbs For Animals

The use of herbs goes back *before* the dawn of human history. Numerous examples have now surfaced of animals using herbs to solve health problems, and many animals have been observed "practicing medicine without a license."

Our Native Americans have a saying: "If you feel sick, reach out your hand." They believe that healing plants grow where they are needed.

Symptoms:

- lethargy
- loss of appetite
- bowel irregularity
- dark urine

The patient lay down most of the day, napping from time to time and taking in no nourishment.

After a period of about eight hours, she began to chew on shoots she painstakingly gathered from a shrub that grows naturally in her vicinity. The shrub is called Veronia amygdalina and was never a part of her diet. In fact, because it was so bitter, it was usually avoided as a foodstuff. However, she chewed the shoots, swallowing the bitter juice and discarding the fiber.

By the next afternoon, although still a bit fatigued, she was eating at regular intervals and her urine and bowel movements were back to normal.

Did she pay her herb doctor for his advice and choice of medicine? No!

The patient in this case was a monkey. A chimpanzee from the Mahale branch and her choice of a healing herb is one example of a sick animal choosing an herb with known medicinal qualities to heal itself. It's no coincidence that African tribes in the vicinity use extracts from the same plant to treat a variety of human problems . . . including treating the very symptoms the chimp was suffering from. They know it can turn your body into a vast germ-slaughtering machine.

Where did the chimp get the knowledge of pharmacology that led her to pick the correct herb for her symptoms?

And why have we lost the ability to "reach out our hands when we feel sick?'

There's another chimp clan living in Gombe National Park. Most of the time they live a normal monkey life. They get up after sunrise, scrounge around for food, make love and then climb a tree to sleep. However, once a month or so they get up earlier than usual and head out as a group. They walk past their favorite fruit trees, on a two-mile trek, to where two members of the sunflower family grow in profusion. We know them as Aspilia mossambicensis and Aspilia pluriseta. What the chimps call them is not known. Very carefully, each chimp examines the leaves looking for unbro-

It's no coincidence that African tribes in the vicinity use extracts from the same plant to treat a variety of human problems. They know it can turn your body into a vast germ-slaughtering machine.

This red sulfur-containing oil has as much anti-cancer activity as other standard chemotherapy agents. How did the chimps found out?

ken ones. Then, with much grimacing and contorting, and with much rolling of the eyes . . . they swallow the leaf whole. This looking, picking, grimacing and swallowing takes most of the morning, after which they slowly trudge home.

Uncharacteristic behavior?

Not for the herbal-aware chimps.

When these leaves were studied, it was determined that they contained an oil now called thiarurbrine-A which kills disease-causing bacteria, fungi and parasitic worms.

Recent studies done on this red sulfur-containing oil shows it to have as much anti-cancer activity in cultured human cervical cells as vincristine and vinblastine, standard chemotherapy agents obtained from another botanical, the periwinkle.

The chimps can't know that.

But they know enough to swallow the leaves unbroken!

Why unbroken? That was a problem to the investigators. Elroy Rodriguez, plant chemist, University of California, Irvine and Harvard anthropologist R.W. Wrangham undertook a chemical analysis of the leaves. They discovered that, in order to be effective against the disease-causing organisms, the oil in the leaves had to be released in the intestines. Of course, during normal passage through the body, the leaves are ruptured and broken, presumably right in the area where they will do the most medicinal good. And unless they were swallowed whole, they would release their power uselessly in the mouth and stomach!

Wow!

How did the chimps find out about the plants and how to take them?

Rx:

- Aspilia leaves #6

Directions:

- Swallow each leaf carefully without breaking.

Dr. Nature.

There's another preserve for chimps in Uganda's Kibala Forest. The sunflower plants do not grow there. However, another plant called Rubia cordifolia grows there in profusion. Chimps have been observed swallowing its leaves whole and Ugandans use the leaves to treat stomach complaints from common to serious conditions.

Howler monkeys in Costa Rica may have discovered a method of choosing the sex of their offspring. When they are pregnant the females eat certain, as yet unidentified, plants which they avoid during the rest of the year. Researchers suspect these plants contain chemicals that change the pH of their vagina, a change that shifts the odds to a male offspring (the more males the female has, the better her position in the tribe).

But herbal wisdom is not limited to monkeys. Bears are known to seek out the herb Ligusticum porteri. This vanilla-scented shrub grows in the Rocky Mountains and the Southwest. The bear digs up the root which he then methodically chews into a pulp. When this root is sufficiently mixed with saliva, he spits it out into his paws and rubs it into his fur.

This herb has a reported use as an insecticide and anti-parasitic agent. The Navaho call the plant, "Bear Medicine," and use it as an insecticide and de-worming herb.

Who told who?

Then there was a pregnant elephant at Tsavo Park in Kenya. Elephants carry for 20 to 22 months, and all during that time this elephant had her routine of walking about ten miles a day and eating her favorite bush plants. Each day she'd walk past trees that were not to her liking. Except that one day when she stopped in front of a particular small tree of the Boraginaceae species. She had passed this tree many times in the almost two years she was pregnant, but this time she examined it very carefully. Her trunk passed up and down, investigating the leaves, the branches and the trunk. She even huffed and puffed at the soil, sampling the earth and the roots. Then she ate the whole tree. Quietly, patiently, she reduced the tree to a denuded

This herb has a reported use as an insecticide and anti-parasitic agent. The Navaho call the plant, "Bear Medicine," and use it as an insecticide and de-worming herb.

skeleton, then ate the skeleton. When she was through, only a depression in the ground hinted at where the tree had been.

Two days later she gave birth to her son.

Coincidence?

Sure. But how come the natives of Kenya use a tea made from the bark of that same species of tree to induce labor?

But we don't have to go so far away to understand the innate herbal wisdom found in animals that we have somehow lost.

Watch your house cat. When she has fur balls, she goes out in the garden and carefully sniffs at the grass before selecting the fronds which appeal to her. Then she eats her medicine until she's able to throw up the fur balls.

Who instructed her?

The Safety Of Herbs And Supplements Vs. Pharmaceuticals

The FDA is rightly concerned with the safety aspects of herbs and restricts the amount of information that is allowed on the label. But, as you can see from the following list, it may be overly concerned about natural products and under-concerned about other products.

The FDA may be overly concerned about natural products and under-concerned about other products.

HERBS	No. of Poisonings 1991
Ginseng (Ren Shen)	0
Echinacea	0
Dandelion	0
Angelica (Dong Gui)	0
Astraguli	0
Rehmanniae	0
Bupleuri	0
Polygoni Multiflori	0
Goldenseal	0
Hawthorn	0
Total	**0**

VITAMIN	No. of Poisonings 1991
Vitamin A	0
Vitamin C	0
Vitamin D	0
Vitamin E	0
Iron	0
Zinc	0
Vitamin B or B-Complex	0
Calcium	0
Magnesuim	0
Potassium	0
Total	**0**

PHARMACEUTICALS*	No. of Poisonings 1991
Analgesics	2669
Antidepressants	517
Antihistamines	412
Antimicrobials	953
Asthma Therapies	257
Cardiovascular Drugs	370
Cough & Cold Preparations	1526
Gastrointestinal Preparations	619
Hormones & Hormone Antagonists	488
Anti-Anxiety/Anti-Psychotics	888
Topicals	1106
Total	**9805**

*Some of the poisonings were considered suicide attempts.
The poison control centers do not differentiate such factors when gathering yearly totals.

Aloe Vera

Happily, scientists are looking at herbs, exploring the folklore that has been the mainstay of "cures" for generations, and even going into the oceans to uncover "superstar" remedies.

What's available to us that we can reach out our hands for and pick up at the local health store?

Let's start with an old friend, aloe vera.

Aloe has enjoyed a reputation as a healing plant for thousands of years. King Solomon used it as a laxative and history books say that Alexander

Let's start with an old friend, aloe vera. It has enjoyed a reputation as a healing plant for thousands of years.

the Great, urged on by Aristotle, conquered the island of Socotra because the plant was plentiful there and he would have a ready supply for his troops. Hippocrates mentions at least 14 medicinal combinations utilizing aloe, and Queen Nefertiti and Cleopatra considered aloe juice among their best cosmetics.

Here's what we already knew about aloe that has been confirmed by science:

Aloe, like garlic, is finding a use in the treatment of cancer.

- It combats inflammation and swelling.
- Its germicidal properties kill bacteria, fungi and possible virus enemies.
- Its anesthetic action eases pain, stings and burns.
- It promotes wound healing.
- It contains chemicals which penetrate the outer layer of skin and cell membranes; this enables it to deliver beneficial compounds deep into your tissue where they can do the most good.

According to Wendell D. Winters, Ph.D., associate professor of microbiology at the University of Texas Health Science Center in San Antonio, no matter what type of external insults you're talking about—cuts, bruises, minor burns or sunburn—aloe will relieve the pain and heal it faster.

John P. Heggers, professor of surgery at the University of Texas at Galveston, believes that aloe can reverse the tissue damage caused by radiation treatment.

Aloe vera helps save skin and limbs if they're frostbitten (*Annals of Emergency Medicine*), it helps heal herpes zoster (shingles), and also helps heal specific types of stomach ulcers. However, although a remarkable herb, these healing qualities have been written about before. It is the new discoveries that have piqued the scientific community.

Aloe, like garlic, is a member of the lily family and, like garlic, it is finding a use in the treatment of cancer. Aloe has been shown to contain phytochemicals called lectins which can activate growth factors inherent in human cells and speed healing. The lectins in aloe stimulate production of cancer-fighting blood cells. A few years ago, Russian scientists evaluated the ability of aloe juice to stop the spread of cancer (metastases). Although it did not stop the main tumor growth, it was able to reduce the frequency of metastases. (Gribel, N.V. and Pashinskii, V.G. Antimetastastic properties of Aloe Juice, *Vopr Onkol*. 1986; 32:38-40)

When shopping for an alóe product look for one that contains at least 50 to 80 percent pure aloe. Products containing less aloe will not be anywhere as effective. In the Pacific Rim, from Australia to Korea, people drink aloe soft drinks, take concentrated aloe juices internally and use liquid and aloe creams externally. They regard aloe as a health food with medicinal values.

In the United States, aloe is accepted as a food supplement without any claims attached but is widely available in most health food stores.

Astragalus

Astragalus (astragalus membranaceus) is the root of a member of the pea family that was used by Chinese doctors for centuries to stimulate a patient's energy. Today, it enjoys the reputation of an adaptogen. Research done in the People's Republic of China has shown that it operates through four main pathways of action.

- On the cellular level, it enhances cell metabolism, delaying the cell's aging, prolonging its life and making it more energy efficient.
- It boosts protein synthesis in the liver with an improvement in nutrition and an increase in energy.
- It stimulates your body's immune system.
- It restores improved functioning to the adrenal cortex, improving metabolism in general.

All in all, it can be said to slam the brakes on the aging of each cell in your body. The cell acts as though it were "young" again; it doesn't develop tumors; and it gives your body two or three times as much energy as before.

In the Pacific Rim, from Australia to Korea, people drink aloe soft drinks, take concentrated aloe juices internally and use liquid and aloe creams externally. They regard aloe as a health food with medicinal values.

The polysaccharides found in astragalus increase the production of interferon and the white blood cells.

Health food stores carry a number of Chinese herbal preparations containing astragalus, usually in combination with other Chinese herbs for their synergistic effect. Follow label directions.

Antistress Astragalus

Dr. Yindi Zhang et al., at China's Nanjing Medical College, tested the effects of two astragalus saponins in immune enhancement and stimulation of stamina and endurance. The research showed that two astragalus saponins, given orally, inhibit suppression of the immune system by cyclophosphamide, and also protect against gamma ray damage to the immune system.

In the endurance, stamina and antistress tests, the researchers showed that mice given these astragalus saponins for ten days (orally) performed better in the swimming test which tests the length of time a mouse can swim before exhaustion, and also increased their resistance to low and high temperatures.

These studies have become standard tests in China of the adaptogenic potential for herbs. The same saponins injected intraperitoneally dramatically increased the level of ascorbic acid in the adrenals.

Astragalus and Viral Heart Disease

In a series of articles in the *Chinese Medical Journal*, doctors at The Shanghai Institute of Cardiovascular Diseases described the overwhelming victory of this anti-germotic, astragalus membranaceus, against the Coxsackie B virus. Among other things, this virus can cause a catastrophic infection of the heart called Coxsackie B viral myocarditis. This disease has become common in China recently and, with dozens of jet liners leaving China every day for America, will soon spread here.

Doctors described the overwhelming victory of this anti-germotic, astragalus, against the virus.

There is currently no drug known to prevent or treat this killer. But, in 1987 Chinese researchers proved that extracts of astragalus literally blew the virus apart, before it could possibly damage heart cells. Yang, Y.Z. et al. *Chinese Medical Journal,* 1987, 107(7):595.)

Following up on this research, the same group has released the results of their latest experiments. In another cultured heart cell experiment, Yuan Wei-long et al. demonstrated that astragalus could reduce cardiac cell damage and changes in electrical activity of heart cells. Heart cells that were already infected were treated with astragalus extract. Within hours, the cells went back to their more regular rhythms, beat more strongly and began repairing the existing cellular damage from the virus infection (*CMJ.* 1990, 103(3): 177-182).

The results of the in vitro experiments were confirmed in another study with Coxsackie B 3 virus-infected mice. Compared with controls, those mice given the Astragalus extract were significantly protected against the effects of the virus-induced heart disease. Both the size and severity of lesions on the heart muscle were reduced by the Astragalus extract, as was the titer or quantity of virus present in the effective heart tissue. The degree of protection was impressive. In untreated controls, 20 percent of the heart muscle was damaged by the viral infection, while in the Astragalus-treated group less than three percent damage resulted from the viral infection. Stated in another way, the Astragalus extract was over 85 percent effective in preventing heart damage from virus infection (*CMJ.* 1990, 103(1):14-18).

Finally, clinical experiments were conducted with human patients suffering from Coxsackie B viral myocarditis, all of whom showed weakened immune systems, as evidenced by depressed natural killer (NK) cell activity. Ten patients were assigned to an Astragalus group and were treated with intramuscular injections of Astragalus extract at a dosage of eight grams per day for three to four months. Another six patients were given "conventional treatment" that consisted of vitamin C, coenzyme A, DNA, and Chinese herbal compound drug Sheng Mai Chong Ji. After therapy,

Chinese researchers proved that extracts of astragalus literally blew the virus apart.

NK activity was tripled in the Astragalus group from 15.6 percent to 44.9 percent.

Also, according to the authors, "the general condition of these patients markedly improved."

Are there side effects when you take these anti-germotics like astragalus? Most certainly! Given their protection, three patients discovered that they "were virtually free from attacks of the common cold and seven had occasional attacks only." In the conventional therapy group "there was no significant change in the NK activity and the clinical condition showed no improvement."

If you take astragalus, it would appear, literally, that it does blow viruses apart the moment they enter your body. Viruses that are so powerful, they tear your heart apart. But they can't touch you now. If you have scars on your heart now — and you can detect them by the fatigue and shortness of breath that are slowly turning you into an invalid — daily doses of this anti-germotic will actually fade them away.

Echinacea
CBS Evening News

On February 17, 1993, the CBS Evening News, in its continuing coverage of alternative medical modalities, featured a piece on echinacea. The news segment began with a brief discussion of the use of supplements, primarily vitamin C, for the prevention of colds and flu. Then they switched to the primary focus of the news story — echinacea. The report noted the popularity of echinacea and its emergence as a popular preventive and treatment for colds and flu. CBS took the viewer to the shelves of a health/natural food store and panned to an array of echinacea products commonly available in these retail outlets. As they explained historical aspects of usage, and noted recent research on the herb that provides a scientific basis for its safety and efficacy, they zoomed in on close-ups of various echinacea

If you have scars on your heart now, daily doses of this anti-germotic will actually fade them away.

products found in the store. The segment also featured a close-up of Christopher Hobb's book, *Echinacea: The Immune Herb.*

Dr. Norman Farnsworth, head of the Program for Collaborative Research in the Pharmaceutical Sciences at the University of Illinois, Chicago, and one of America's best-known medicinal plant experts was interviewed by CBS. Farnsworth indicated that research out of Germany suggested a pharmacological basis for the efficacy of echinacea.

Echinacea and the Immune System

The primary modern use for echinacea preparations in Europe is as a non-specific immunostimulant. Echinacea is used to enhance or "stimulate" the body's own resistance against infections, especially in the prevention of colds and flu. If taken at the first sign of a cold or flu or uncontrollable coughing, in small, frequent doses every two to three hours for the first two days, it often helps to mobilize the body's own resistance to the condition and stops the symptoms dead in their tracks, eliminating any further need for antibiotics.

Immunostimulants are agents that stimulate the immune system in a non-specific manner. An increase in phagocytosis (by macophages and granulocytes) is an important factor in immunostimulation. Non-specific immunostimulatory actions fade relatively quickly requiring repeated dosage to sustain effect. Since the late 1970's a number of studies have explored the immune-system-stimulating potential of echinacea preparations.

Reuter, H.D. Phytotherapy: when the immune system requires help. *Munch. Med. Wschr.* 133: 46-50, 1991.

In another of a series of outstanding articles by Prof. Reuter, he notes that in the last 30 years much research has been dedicated to why certain plant substances are able to stimulate the immune system. Prof. Reuter acknowledges that the answer to this question has been a difficult one, given the fact that plants are complex combinations of numerous naturally-

> *If taken at the first sign of a cold or flu, it often helps stop the symptoms dead in their tracks, eliminating any further need for antibiotics.*

"Giant eating cells" start our bodies' destruction of bacterial or viral debris that the body has targeted for elimination.

occuring chemicals. However, one answer as to why certain plant substances are immunostinulatory lies in the concept of polysaccharides.

Polysaccharides, as previously stated, are long complex chains of sugar molecules that are distinct from other types of sugars like lactose (milk sugar), sucrose (table sugar), and glucose (blood sugar in animals). This inherent uniqueness in structure is comparable to building a house or skyscraper. Although both use similar building materials, the final outcome is very different. Polysaccharides are simply the skyscrapers of sugar.

The list of herbs containing these polysaccharides is a distinguished one and includes the following examples: Shiitake mushroom (lentinan edodes), marigold (calendula officinalis), marshmallow (althea officinalis), saw palmetto (sabal serrulata), Siberian ginseng (eleutherococcus senticosus), and of course purple cornflower (echinacea purpurea).

Echinacea, as Prof Reuter points out, is one of the world's most extensively researched immunostimulatory herbs. Echinacea's polysaccharides (arabinogalactans) work primarily by stimulating our macrophage-mediated defense system. Macrophages or "giant eating cells" start our bodies' destruction of, for example, bacterial or viral debris that the body has targeted for elimination. However, these macrophages do more than just provide a sophisticated clean-up service.

Pharmacological research shows that echinacea preparations help stimulate the body's own defense system of cellular immunity. Echinacea works primarily through stimulating cellular or non-specific immunity, as opposed to specific immunity, such as that produced by antibodies reacting to a specific antigen (which is how vaccines work).

Echinacea seems to stimulate a complement of non-specific mechanisms such as phagosytosis by leukocytes (various types of white blood corpuscles which act as scavengers in order to help combat infections). Components of echinacea inhibit hyaluronidase, an enzyme involved in the infection process. Various components have mild bacteriostatic and fungistatic activity — helping to allay the spread of pathogens, rather than killing them outright as an antibiotic would do. By increasing fibroblasts (cells involved in the development of connective tissue), it helps to stimulate new tissue development. Studies on properdin levels have shown that this serum protein complex, which helps to activate various aspects of the immune system, is increased by echinacea extracts, providing a further mechanism for its immunostimulatory action. Studies have also shown that echinacea may also act by stimulating increased production of interferon (an important component of immune function) by macrophages. In addition, echinacea has anti-inflammatory activity).

When purchasing echinacea, look for a product containing both water-soluble principles and alcohol-soluble principles. The label will tell you if it is a complete extract of these two principles. The product will be most effective if taken four times a day at the first sign of a cold or infection. If you prefer the liquid, take a full teaspoon in juice since the taste is pretty strong.

Echinacea is available at most health food stores and drugstores. Many people report best results when it is taken in combination with vitamin C.

Feverfew is fast becoming one of the most sought-after alternative medicines for pain relief.

Got a Headache?
Chew On A Plant . . . Not Aspirin

Not any old plant, Tanacetum parthenium.

At the botanical garden?

No, at your health food store.

Also known as feverfew, it is fast becoming one of the most sought-after alternative medicines for pain relief. Alternative medicine is a 20th century term which refers to herbal or homeopathic medicine, acupuncture, osteopathy, vitamins and minerals, etc., despite the fact that these treatments have been with us for decades and even for thousands of years. To be brutally honest, orthodox medicine, which has been around only a few hundred years should really be called "alternative medicine." But,

To be brutally honest, orthodox medicine, which has been around only a few hundred years should really be called "alternative medicine."

since the advent of World War II, based on the undeniable impact of penicillin, folk medicine was pushed far into the background. However, due to the considerable impact now being felt from certain herbs, and the fact that synthetic medicine with its considerable side effects has not wrought the miracle changes heralded, a renaissance of folk medicine is imminent.

Witness the official Canadian acceptance of a feverfew product made by a British firm intended to help migraine sufferers. This is a good sign to those involved in the promotion of natural remedies.

"Official recognition of the potential of feverfew in migraine prevention will likely serve as an incentive to further clinical evaluation of traditional remedies," said D.V.C. Awang, Ph.D., head of the Natural Products Bureau of Drug Research, Health Branch, Health and Welfare, Canada.

The approval allows the product to make the claim and be sold as a non-prescription drug that prevents migraine headaches.

Approval of the feverfew claim was based on two clinical trials conducted in the United Kingdom in 1985 and 1988 at the University of Nottingham (placebo-controlled, double-blind, cross-over and randomized study).

The study utilized freeze-dried and air-dried feverfew leaf. 125 mg containing at least 0.2 percent parthenolide is the recommended preventive treatment for migraine. It is the rough equivalent of two medium-sized feverfew leaves daily.

Because feverfew has also been used as a diaphoretic, to lower fever, scientists hypothesized that the method of action on the body might be similar to aspirin. The active ingredients in feverfew inhibit the production of certain prostaglandins, thus blocking or reducing inflammatory conditions in your body, determining how much blood is distributed to tissues. This is important, for it is the widening and narrowing of blood vessels in the brain that have been linked to migraine headaches; and the inflammatory process itself causes pain, swelling, and even disfiguring of joints and other tissues which this can prevent. The narrowing of blood vessels reduces the blood supply to certain parts of the brain. Expansion or dilation of the vessels can cause the feeling of fullness or pressure and pounding in your brain that makes many headache sufferers consider suicide.

Parthenolides inhibit leukotrienes, slow-acting substances that stimulate allergic reactions. They also inhibit other substances called amines which are known to increase in the brain during the early stages of a migraine attack. Certain foods contain similar amines and are considered to be "trigger" foods — foods like coffee, chocolate and some fried foods — so the parthenolides in feverfew let you eat these foods again without paying the price in pain.

And, unlike aspirin, feverfew has few side effects.

If you are one of the people who does not benefit from feverfew, there are other herbal plans for you. Dilute 10 drops of lavender oil in 25 cc of almond or wheat germ oil. Mix well and at the first sign of an attack, gently massage into your temples. Then make a tea of 1 teaspoon of lavender flower and one teaspoon of vervain to 1 cup of water.

Or, try taking 2 cc of tincture of Jamaican dogwood 3 times a day. Both available at your health food store.

Feverfew blocks the inflammation that can cause the feeling of pressure and pounding that makes many headache sufferers consider suicide.

More About Garlic And Onions — Antioxidant, Anti-Tumor, Cardiovascular Action And Anti-Ulcer Effects

Garlic continues to be one of the most intensively studied of medicinal plants. With most research focusing on anticarcinogenic and cardiovascular protective effects of garlic, researchers at China's Shandong Academy of Medical Science reported the effects of allicin, one of garlic's least stable compounds, as an antioxidant. They documented an antioxidant effect of allicin, and also a possible mechanism for this action. Allicin increased the levels of two important antioxidant enzymes in the blood: catylase and

Topical application of the compounds from garlic significantly increased the survival rate.

glutathione peroxidase. This confirmed the antioxidant and free-radical scavenging potential of allicin.

Meanwhile, American researchers at South Dakota State University studied the effects of garlic and onion oil in preventing skin tumors. The study focused on two oil soluble compounds from garlic, diallyl sulfide and diallyl disulfide, in protecting mice against carcinogen-induced skin tumors. Topical application of the compounds significantly inhibited formation of tumors and increased the survival rate. "These findings support earlier evidence that these naturally occurring compounds may be useful for the chemoprevention of certain types of tumors."

Japanese researchers explored the sulfur compounds in aged garlic extract, a popular deodorized form of garlic. They found five sulfur compounds which inhibited lipid peroxidation in the liver, that is, they are antioxidants, preventing a reaction which is considered to be one of the main features of aging in liver cells. The sulfur compounds themselves "appear to be approximately 1000 times more potent in antioxidant activity than the crude aged garlic extract."

Scientists at Northwestern University (Evanston, Illinois) studied the anticarcinogenic action of diallyl sulfide, reporting their results in *Cancer Letters*.

This research study demonstrated that diallyl sulfide is effective as an anticarcinogen, while serving as a test of a "novel cost-effective strategy for the rapid identification of tissue-specific anticarcinogens and a quantitative assessment of their efficacy."

Cardiovascular effects have long been studied for garlic, especially its effects in lowering blood cholesterol, possibly inhibiting atherosclerosis. Scientists at Venezuela's Laboratory of Thrombosis Experimentation demonstrated the effect of ajoene from garlic in preventing clot formation produced by hidden viral damage in your arteries and veins.

The chemical is known to be a potent antiplatelet compound which is isolated from alcoholic extracts of garlic. Ajoene is known to reversibly inhibit platelet aggregation (leading to clot formation), but this research focused specifically on clot formation caused by mildly or severely damaged blood vessel walls. In this type of injury, turbulence in the arteries can cause platelet aggregation and clot formation, which can result in heart attack or stroke. The experiment was designed to mimic the conditions of blood flow in small and medium-sized arteries by varying the velocity of the blood. The compound was found effective in both conditions, and authors suggest that it may be useful in emergency treatment to prevent clot formation produced by vascular damage.

Finally, a new study at Chile's Concepcion University reported that an extract of garlic bulbs inhibited cardiovascular function in dogs, suggesting a "beta-blocker" mechanism. The extract was made from fresh garlic homogenized in twice its weight of water, heated for 5 minutes and concentrated to 10 times its strength by evaporation. The resulting concentrate was purified by dialysis, and administered by injection (i.v.). It produced a rapid drop in blood pressure and heart rate. The effect on heart rate was confirmed on isolated heart muscle, decreasing the strength and frequency of muscle contractions.

This potent antiplatelet compound from garlic may be useful in emergency treatment to prevent clot formation.

More Anti-Cancer Evidence for Garlic

German scientists K. Scharfenberg et al. reported in a recent issue of *Cancer Letters* on their experiments with cytotoxic effects of two garlic components against 3 different cell lines. Cytotoxic agents are lethal to living cells and the goal in researching them is to find compounds which are more lethal to cancer cells than to normal cells. This in vitro experiment used cultured cells including normal human body cells (fibroblasts) and a malignant cell line derived from "Burkitt Lymphoma." There were several interesting discoveries from this experiment. First, the test found that it takes about three hours for the garlic compounds to be incorporated into the cell, but that their effect was almost immediate once they had entered the cell. The chemical compound ajoene, which is a breakdown product

It was twice as toxic to malignant cells as to normal cells.

of allicin, was about twice as active as allicin itself and is more stable than allicin, which gradually decomposes. Most importantly though, ajoene was twice as toxic to malignant cells as to normal cells, which greatly increases its potential therapeutic usefulness. The authors also point out that the difference in sensitivity of malignant cells compared to normal cells is in accord with other evidence indicating that ajoene is non-irritating to the skin and even to the eyes. (Scharfenberg, K. et al. 1990, *Cancer Letters* 53:103-108.)

Anti-Ulcer Effect of Garlic

Along with numerous other health benefits of garlic, there is now evidence of an anti-ulcer effect. Recent studies at the Catholic university Medical College in Seoul, Korea, focused on the protective effect of two major garlic compounds, allicin and deallyl disulfide, in protecting the stomach against damage from ethyl (grain) alcohol. This study, by Sok Won Han et al., showed that diallyl disulfide, a breakdown product of the pungent ingredient of garlic, protected the stomach lining against ethanol-induced damage. The results of this study were that the garlic compound "completely protected the stomach against mucosal damage induced by absolute ethanol."

Since it had already been determined that garlic and its chemical compounds do not decrease the amount of stomach acid produced, this study sought to determine the mechanism by which garlic might protect against alcohol-induced damage. The probable mechanism was found when the researchers measured an increase in the production of prostaglandins by garlic-stimulated stomach cells. Prostaglandins are important chemical mediators of inflammation and pain. Apparently, the mild irritation of the garlic compound triggers a protective reaction which decreases subsequent damage by the alcohol. (Sok Won Han et al., 1990, *Bulletin of Clinical Research* CMC 18(2):223-236.)

Immune Stimulation

Though not as well documented, garlic seems to have immunostimu-lant effects, acting as a nonspecific stimulant to the immune system. It increases phagocytosis, by which invading organisms and abnormal cells are eliminated from the body. It also causes a dramatic increase in natural killer (NK) cell activity, which at least partially explains its anti-cancer, antiviral and antimicrobial effects. Experiments have shown that one com-ponent of garlic, called diallyl sulfide, can completely inhibit the induction of esophageal cancer by nitrosamines. These potent carcinogens are con-sidered the major cause of this type of cancer, and among the most potent carcinogens overall. The garlic compound actually reduced metabolism of the nitrosamine by the liver, a unique anti-carcinogenic activity.

Rotzsch, W., Richter, V. et al: Postprandial lipemia under treatment with Allium sativum: Controlled double-blind study in healthy volunteers with reduced HDL2-cholesterol levels. *Arzneim-Forsch Drug Res* 42: 1223-7, 1992.

The effectiveness of a standardized garlic powder preparation on high triglyceride levels after intake of a standardized fatty test meal containing 100 g butter was analyzed in a randomized placebo-controlled double-blind study. 24 volunteers with HDL2-cholesterol concentrations in plasma of less than 10 mg/dl (men) and 15 mg/dl (women) participated in the study. The treatment group received 300 mg of the garlic powder three times daily for six weeks. The after-meal increase of triglycerides was clearly reduced under garlic medication as compared to placebo treatment (values for triglycerides were 35% lower in the garlic group). Fasting triglycerides after the six week study period were also lower for the garlic group and HDL2-cholesterol (good cholesterol!) increased significantly in this group also.

The triglyceride and cholesterol-lowering effect of concentrated garlic powder products continues to be supported by clinical research. In com-bination with nutrients like niacin and chromium, as well as a healthy diet

Garlic also causes a dramatic increase in natural killer cell activity, which partially explains its anti-cancer, antiviral and anti-microbial effects.

These garlic products represent a safe and effective tool to prevent high triglyceride and cholesterol levels.

and regular exercise, these garlic products represent a safe and effective tool to either treat or prevent high triglyceride and cholesterol levels.

Garlic Fights Nitrosamine Formation . . .

Nitrosamines and related toxic N-nitroso compounds induce cancer through the formation of adducts — their tight chemical bonds to DNA. But, at least in rats, adding high concentrations of garlic powder to the diet can greatly quash the formation of such adducts, according to nutritionists at Pennsylvania State University in University Park.

John A. Milner and his colleagues exposed their animals for 2 or 3 weeks to chemicals known to generate nitrosamines in the gut — and subsequent liver or mammary cancers. Over the same period, some of the animals consumed large amounts of garlic: 2 to 4 percent of their diet by weight. The treated rodents didn't seem to object to the heavy seasoning, since they ate as much food as rats offered garlic-free chow.

The big difference appeared in the number of adducts the rats developed, Milner and his coworkers report in the Feb. 8 *Carcinogenesis*. Penn State's cuisine produced a drop of some 40 to more than 80 percent — depending on the amount of garlic in the diet — in the predominant liver adducts that form in animals administered the nitrosamine or nitrosamine precursors used in this experiment. Garlicky chow also produced a dose-dependent reduction of 55 to 69 percent in mammary adducts associated with another nitrosamine.

Milner's team suspects that some of garlic's anti-cancer benefits also stem from the ability of its organic sulfur compounds to break down and detoxify nitrosamines.

. . . As Do Tomatoes and Other Produce

Cornell University food scientists published data showing that eating green peppers, pineapples, carrots, strawberries — and especially tomatoes — can suppress the formation of nitrosamines in humans. Though these fruits and vegetables all contain vitamin C, which can derail the reaction that produces nitrosamines, the researchers began looking for additional blockers when they determined that each food's nitrosamine-inhibiting potency was greater than could be accounted for by its vitamin C alone.

In *Agricultural and Food Chemistry*, Cornell's Michael A. Helser and Joseph H. Hotchkiss identified two new nitrosamine blockers — p-coumaric and chlorogenic acids. Together, these phenols provide about 35 to 40 percent of a juiced tomato's nitrosamine-inhibiting activity. Though these compounds occur in many types of produce, green coffee beans constitute one of the riches sources of chlorogenic acids.

Overall, Helser and Hotchkiss found that the ascorbate (vitamin C) fraction of a tomato contains about half the fruit's nitrosamine-inhibiting activity. However, their data also suggests that because pure vitamin C appears to account for only about one-quarter of the inhibition associated with a tomato's ascorbate fraction, even the vitamin C portion appears to carry potent, as-yet-unmasked nitrosamine blockers.

... And Onions

Dorsch, W., Schneider, E. et al: Anti-inflammatory effects of onions: Inhibition of chemotaxis of human polymorphonuclear leukocytes by thiosulfinates and cepanes. *Int Arch Allergy Appl Immunol* 92:39-42,1990.

Seven different synthetic thiosulfinates and cepane-and/or thiosulfinate-rich onion extracts were found to inhibit in vitro the chemotaxis of human granulocytes induced by formyl-methionine-leucine-phenylalanine in a dose-dependent manner and were found to be more active than prednisolone. The anti-inflammatory properties of onion extracts are related, at least in part, to the inhibition of inflammatory cell influx by thiosulfinates and cepanes.

The authors of this study have previously shown the ability of thiosulfinates, the sulfur-containing active principles of onions, to inhibit both the cyclooxygenase and lipoxygenase pathways of arachadonic acid

Cornell University food scientists published data showing that eating green peppers, pineapples, carrots, strawberries — and especially tomatoes — can suppress the formation of nitrosamines in humans.

The cure rate of anti-germotics like garlic now approaches 100 percent, even against the super microbes and viruses that eat antibiotics for lunch.

metabolism. They also have the ability to inhibit histamine release and have inhibited bronchial asthma in animals challenged with inhalant allergens and platelet-activating factor. Cepanes were later shown to have similar effect. The above findings relate directly to late-phase allergic reactions.

It is interesting that syrup made from onions and honey was used as part of a management scheme for asthma in many home-medicine cabinets. Also, an extremely useful tool for asthma is the use of onion poultices to the chest — especially for children. With a renewed increase in the use of prednisone for asthma, increased effort should be made by schools specializing in natural product research to study onion extracts as a potentially more effective, safe, and inexpensive alternative.

Garlic Studied for Obesity and Meningitis

Researchers at the Haemorraeology unit of the Munich University have found that garlic is a fat-reducing agent. A clinical study carried out on 20 patients showed that ten out of twenty using garlic tablets had lower cholesterol levels. Another study written up in the official Chinese medical journal claimed that an extract of garlic is a cheap and most effective remedy for meningitis. "Whilst garlic extract provided nearly 82 percent cure, the currently used modern drug, Amphetericin, cured only 15 percent of the cases." The study further asserts that garlic lowers blood pressure, blood sugar levels in diabetic patients, and cures some types of cancer (tumors) besides being an excellent intestinal antiseptic. (*BEPHA Bulletin*, July 86.)

The cure rate of these anti-germotics (like garlic) now approaches 100 percent, even against the super microbes and viruses that eat antibiotics for lunch.

Ginseng

Ginseng was first described in one of the earliest herbal classics, which reports that ginseng is "sweet" in nature and that it has a therapeutic action related to the spleen, stomach, and lungs. The old literature says that ginseng's principal effects nourish the important organs, soothe the mind, stop palpitation due to fright, improve eyesight, and can even induce resuscitation. It is even reported to stop diabetes and improve memory.

Chinese friends say that ginseng invigorates "Qi" which refers to mobility and metabolic function of the body. So "deficiency of qi" means that the function of the body is weak, signs of which would be: weak breath, pulse too fast or too slow, bad sleep and digestion, weak sexual function, and fatigue.

The main action of ginseng is invigorating qi of the lungs for "free" breathing, and better oxygen flow of red blood cells — all of which brings your health status to a new level.

Scientific researchers have also proved that ginseng has the following actions:

1. It is capable of stimulating the cerebral cortex and of regulating and inhibiting metabolic actions. It is an instant shot of energy, even stronger than caffeine, and no letdown later.

2. It enhances the body's ability against antagonists, so that it increases survival duration. It helps the body resist poisons, such as lead, benzene and phenols.

3. It influences internal secretion by improving the integrity of the adrenal glands, thyroid gland, and thymus gland.

4. It influences metabolism by regulating the glycemic (blood sugar) reactions, and by promoting the manufacture of protein and nucleic acids (RNA and DNA).

5. It enhances the immune system, strengthening the ability to resist diseases and foreign bodies.

There are more than 1,000 research papers validating the benefits of ginseng.

Ever since early in the 1970's when ginseng invaded the United States, the impact of the world's largest and most highly-evolved system of herbal

Ginseng's principal effects nourish the important organs, soothe the mind, stop palpitation due to fright, and improve eyesight. It is even reported to stop diabetes and improve memory.

> *When conditions caused by compromised immunity and cancers are increasing, these herbs are being investigated for promises discovered hundreds of years ago. Some even feel, without these super-herbs, your immune system simply cannot function properly.*

medicine has been gaining respect in the United States. First there was ginseng, then we began to learn there were other super-herbs in the Oriental pharmacy. It is appropriate that when conditions caused by compromised immunity and cancers are increasing, herbs like astragalus, and schisandra are being investigated for promises discovered hundreds of years ago. Some even feel, without these super-herbs, your immune system simply cannot function properly.

Siberian ginseng (Eleutherococcus senticosus) belongs to the botanical family Araliaceae, and is a relative of Chinese/Korean ginseng (Panax ginseng). It has been known primarily as an adaptogenic herb (ability to increase resistance to stress and provide a balancing effect regardless of the condition — either excess or deficiency) until 1987 when a German clinical study (*Arzneim-Forsch Drug Research,* Vol. 37, p. 1193-1196) suggested that it was able to stimulate a number of aspects of the immune system. In particular T-lymphocytes and T-lymphocytes helper cells which trigger your body's response aginst infection. Without them, your immune system cannot function properly.

In a Korean study, rats were given a carcinogen with four food substances: red pepper, salt, a spice mixture, and ginseng extract. After a 40 week trial period, the impact on cancers of the intestinal tract was tabulated. The results were dramatic:

DIET ADDITIVE	PERCENTAGE OF ANIMALS WITH TUMORS
Salt	61.9
Red Peppers	57.0
Spices	14.8
Ginseng	3.4

All ginseng can be of great value. There is a variety of American Ginseng (Panax quinquefolius) and Indian Ginseng Ashwagandha (Withania somnifera). The Indian Ginseng is among several plants mentioned in the renowned Ayurvedic text *Charaka Samhita* (1,000 B.C.). However, it took until 1965 to be widely recognized, when researcher S.M. Kupchan demonstrated that the herb had antitumor activity (*Journal of the American Chemistry Society*, Vol. 87, 1965).

More Than Ginsenosides

Recent research on panax ginseng conducted by the Oriental Medicine Research Center, Kitasato Institute, Japan, investigated the protective activity of ginseng polysaccharides against gastric ulcers induced by ethanol (drinking alcohol). Alcohol is known to be one of the most damaging substances to which we expose our stomach lining. It is, in fact, one of only a few substances which can penetrate the lining of the stomach and hence cause damage. A polysaccharide fraction from panax ginseng was found to strongly inhibit gastric damage induced by ethanol. This activity was comparable to that of the synthetic pharmaceutical agent, sucralfate, at the same dose.

Previous research had shown anti-ulcer effects of ginseng saponins (ginsenosides). However, here the protective effects reported were not due to saponins, which had been removed from the fractions active in this test. It is not clear whether these polysaccharides may produce an enhanced, synergistic effect when used in combination with saponins. This research points to the clear probability that whole ginseng is more effective in protecting against gastric damage than isolated ginseng saponins. (X.B. Sun et al. (Jan. 1991), *Journal of Ethnopharmacology* 31 (1): 101-107.)

Alcohol is known to be one of the most damaging substances to which we expose our stomach lining. But, panax ginseng was found to strongly inhibit gastric damage induced by ethanol (drinking alcohol).

New Immunostimulants From Japanese Ginseng

Osamu Tanaka is one of the best known names in Japanese medicinal research. Much of the recent research on ginseng, and especially on the chemistry of ginseng, has been carried out by Tanaka's group at the Institute of Pharmaceutical Sciences of Hiroshima University School of Medicine. In 1987 this group reported the presence of immune-stimulating polysaccharides in sanchi ginseng (panax notoginseng). In October 1989, the researchers K. Ohtani et al. reported for the first time on two polysaccha-

New research in India explores the effects of an extract of the fresh leaf of gotu kola on learning and memory.

rides from panax japonicus which stimulate the immune system in mice. As with the earlier experiments on sanchi (also called tienchi) ginseng, the extracts tested were first treated to remove the saponins (ginsenosides) which have long been considered the most active constituents of the ginsengs. The two polysaccharides were then extracted with hot water and thoroughly analyzed for chemical identity.

Immune stimulation was tested by the well-known carbon clearance test, which measures the speed with which a mouse can clear injected carbon particles from its blood. Both polysaccharides from panax japonicus significantly increased the clearance rate and both outperformed the positive control zymosan. One of the Japanese names of Japanese ginseng is "tochiba-ninjin." From this name, the names of the two new polysaccharides were derived. They were called tochibanan A and B; the former with a molecular weight of 23,000 — around the same size as the actives in astragalus, and the more active compound B, with molecular weight of 40,000. The structure of the first compound is elucidated in the article, and a possible structure for tochibanan B is proposed. *Chem. Pharm. Bull.*, 37(10), 2587-2591 (1989).

Although ginseng is the best known of the Chinese herbs, the list of beneficial herbs used in China is a long one. Astragalus, schisandra, dong-quai, licorice, fo-ti, ginger, garlic, ephedra, just to name a few.

Gotu Kola

Gotu kola (Centella asiatica) is now being used in Europe for its effects on mental function. New research in India explores the effects of an aqueous (water) extract of the fresh leaf on learning and memory. Gotu kola has sometimes been confused in the popular and medical media with cola nut, a source of caffeine and cola beverages. The unrelated Indian food and medicinal plant called gotu kola contains no caffeine and is said to be the favorite food of the Indian elephant. Also known as Indian pennywort, this is a low-growing herb fond of moist and shady conditions.

The recent research follows on reports that centella improves memory and helps overcome negative effects of stress and fatigue. Surprisingly, other research shows an alcohol extract has sedative effects on rats. Two studies have shown benefits to mentally retarded children, improving their IQ and behavior. The current study focused on one of the proposed mechanisms of activity, an effect on the neurotransmitters norepinephrine, dopamine and serotonin. The extract used was made by grinding fresh leaves with a small amount of water and expressing the extract. One ml of the extract corresponded to .38 g of fresh leaves. However, dosages cited in the report are in terms of the fresh leaves. No toxicity was noted at any dosage level, from 0.1 to 16.0 g/kg of body weight. The highest dose used would be equivalent to 1120 g (nearly 2.5 pounds for an average 154-pound human). This is excellent documentation of the safety of the plant, which has long been used as a food in much of Asia.

Test results showed an impressive improvement in memory in rats, which were treated daily with the extract (orally) for 14 days before the experiment. The memory of learned behavior in the rats treated with centella skyrocketed 3 to 60 times better than that in control animals. This correlated with a decrease in all the neurotransmitters in the treated animals. This indicates the chemicals (biogenic amines) are involved in learning and memory. The authors conclude, "In summary, the results of the present study prove that C. asiatica improves learning and memory process." (Nalini, K. et al., "Effect of Centella asiatica fresh leaf aqueous extract on learning and memory and biogenic amine turnover in albino rats." *Fitoterapia*, 1992,63(3):232/237.)

Green Tea

The Chinese herbal system is more complex than simply drinking herb tea . . .

Unless it's Green Tea!

The recent research reports that centella improves memory and helps overcome negative effects of stress and fatigue.

Science has uncovered a modern secret the Chinese have known about for centuries. This substance prevents many types of cancer.

Science has uncovered a modern secret the Chinese have known about for centuries. This "brand new" substance prevents many types of cancer in laboratory animals.

It is non-toxic, pleasant and easy to take and, it's not expensive.

The "brand new" substance is green tea, one of the most popular beverages in Asia. Tea has long been considered "that excellent and by All Physicians approved China drink." (1658).

Doctors began the present study when they sought to understand why, when the Japanese have the highest smoking rate, they also have the lowest lung cancer rate in the developed world.

It's a fact, Japanese men have less than one-third the lung cancer of their American counterparts.

This does not mean that you can continue to smoke cigarettes if you drink green tea. It means that there is something in that beverage that can be protective.

Green tea is unfermented. The more common black tea is fermented and Oolong is a mixture of the two. In the late 1980's, Japanese scientists reported that they had isolated a substance from green tea that was able to lower cholesterol and inhibited the growth of cancer. (Chisaka, T. et al. "The effect of crude drugs on experimental hypercholesteremia: mode of action of (-)- epigallocatechin gallate in tea leaves." *Chem Pharm Bull* (Tokyo) 1988; 227-33.

The chemical, shortened to EGCG, was shown to inhibit tumors of the skin and the gastrointestinal tract of experimental mice.

In August of 1991, at the Fourth Chemical Congress of North America, scientists reported that mice given EGCG developed far less lung cancer, and in mice specially bred to develop liver cancer, the tumors would just not appear when they drank this remarkable tea.

According to Dr. Fujiki of the National Cancer Center Research Institute in Tokyo, the average tea lover in Japan ingests about one gram of EGCG daily. Dr. Fujiki said green tea cannot prevent cancer, but it's the cheapest and most practical method for cancer prevention available to the general public.

Green tea may prevent cancer in four ways by:

- Neutralizing cancer-causing ingredients
- Protecting cells against mutation from cancer-causing agents.
- Protecting against free radical damage.
- Protecting against ionizing radiation.

Green tea is available as a tea or in tablets made of powdered leaves. Both are available at health food stores.

Drink a cup with meals, it may save your life!

Another Reason To Drink Green Tea

"Every time you eat a sweet," Isao Kubo's grandmother used to say, "drink green tea." Though Kubo failed to heed her advice, he now acknowledges that he should have. An organic chemist, Kubo reported data last week demonstrating that flavor compounds in the Japanese brew can kill Streptococcus mutans — bacteria that help cause dental caries — and can, therefore, take the damage out of eating sweets. The rule is simplicity itself: for one sweet, take one sip of green tea.

The tea's cavity-fighting potential, confirmed roughly 10 years ago, first appeared to trace back to water-soluble compounds, largely tannins, that can halt S. mutans' production of glucans. These sticky materials bind acid-generating bacteria to teeth. However, a cup of tea did not appear to contain enough glucan inhibitors to account for its anticariogenic activity. So Kubo turned to the tea's hexanes — oily, flora-scented, water-insoluble compounds that give the drink its distinctive flavor.

At least nine of the 10 most abundant flavor compounds in green tea also inhibit glucan production, Kubo's team at the University of California, Berkeley, now reports. Moreover, when certain of these hexanes accompany one another, as they do in the tea, they can kill the microbes — and at far lower levels than required to shut down glucan production. For

The rule is simplicity itself: for one sweet, take one sip of green tea.

It can add 20 to 30 healthy years to your life. Because of its ability to rout infectious bacteria, it prevents them from causing the scars and collapses we call old age.

instance, even at 1,600 parts per million (ppm), caryophyllene alone exhibits no activity against the microbe. But when it accompanies 200 ppm of indole (half of that hexane's bacteria-inhibiting does), a mere 6.25 ppm of caryophyllene kills S. mutans.

Nor are the hexanes' antimicrobial abilities restricted to S. mutans. Kubo found they devastated every killer he tested them against: two molds, three yeasts and eight bacteria, including some responsible for gastrointestinal disease and acne.

What if you don't like green tea? Its active hexanes also occur naturally in coriander, sage and thyme and as approved additives in ice creams, candy, chewing gum and baked goods. In the future, Kubo envisions green tea toothpastes and dental rinses.

Schisandra

Schisandra strengthens reaction time and nervous reflexes.

Fo-Ti (Polygonum multiflrum) is called ho-shou-wu in China and is considered magical in its power to promote longevity. It can add 20 to 30 healthy, vigorous, disease-free years to your life. How can it do this? Because of its ability to rout infectious bacteria. It prevents them from causing the scars and collapses we call old age.

Schisandra is a primary adaptogen with particular restorative power for the nervous system. Its action upon the immune system is noteworthy since it stimulates worn-out immune systems to spring into action becoming devastating, never-ending germ-killing machines. So potent they can even squelch cancer cells, if they should arise in your body.

There are a number of companies converting Chinese herbal formulas into acceptable supplemental formulas. Unfortunately, they cannot spell out on the label what they are to be used for. Your local health food store may be able to advise the suggested use or steer you to a professional who is familiar with Chinese herbology.

Silymarin

Muzes, G., Deak, G. et al: Effect of the bioflavonoid silymarin on the in vitro activity and expression of superoxide dismutase. *Acta Physiol Hungarica* 78:3-9,1991.

Superoxide dismutase (SOD) activity and expression of the red blood cells and lymphocytes of patients suffering from chronic alcoholic liver disease and those of healthy controls were investigated after in vitro (test tube) incubation with silymarin (Legalon). It was concluded that silymarin treatment in a concentration achievable by in vivo (in humans or animals) treatment (10mcg/ml) significantly increased the SOD activity of both the red blood cells and lymphocytes of patients with liver disease. The results further support the ability of silymarin to enhance antioxidant protection of cells and therefore inhibit free radical damage.

Most of the previous research on the antioxidant activity of silymarin has focused on its ability to both increase and spare glutathione, particularly in liver cells (Valenzuela, A. et al: *Planta Medica* 55:420-2.1989). This study expands this antioxidant activity to SOD production also. In addition to glutathione depletion in the liver, SOD activity has been found to be compromised systemically in patients with alcoholic liver disease. This is probably due to toxic end-products of free radical damage in the liver spreading systemically. These results indicate a dramatic rise in SOD levels in both red blood cells and lymphocytes in patients with alcoholic liver disease.

Silymarin continues to grow in stature as one of the plant kingdom's most powerful antioxidants.

Silymarin continues to grow in stature as one of the plant kingdom's most powerful antioxidants.

Suma Cum Laude

First there was ginseng. Then there was pau d' arco. Now comes a new herbal adaptogen, Pfaffia Paniculata (Martius) Kuntze, also known as suma. Found in the rain forests of Brazil, this amaranth-family member is

□

*Suma
has been used
for three
centuries
as a tonic,
aphrodisiac,
and treatment
for diabetes,
tumors and
skin problems.*

being hailed by some researchers as a natural immune-enhancer which can be beneficial in the treatment of some types of cancer, anemia, bronchitis, fatigue, impotence and other maladies.

While most claims for suma still need to be verified through double-blind, placebo-controlled studies in the U.S., it is evident from the research to date that this herb will soon contend for the number one spot in popularity with herb enthusiasts. Indeed, the "Brazilian ginseng" is quickly making a name for itself.

Like pau d' arco, suma is an immune-enchancer, fitting into the category of remedies which help us adapt to new stresses and restore natural immune resistance. Pharmacologists and herbalists call the herbs in this category adaptogens.

Origin

Suma has been used in the Amazon for at least three centuries as a tonic, aphrodisiac, and as a treatment for diabetes, tumors and skin problems. The herb became popular in the Japanese community in Brazil, who first gave it the name "Brazilian ginseng" because of its energizing and rejuvenating properties. This "ginseng," pfaffia paniculata, has nothing to do with imported ginseng: botanically, their vegetable families are quite different. Pfaffia belongs to the Amaranthaceae family while most ginsengs belong to the Araliaceae family.

Research

Eventually, researchers in Japan at the Rohto Pharmaceutical Company, Bunri University, and Hokuriku University began to analyze suma. The first chemical work dealing with the composition of pfaffia paniculata was published in 1983 by Professor Takemoto of the Bunri University. After various research projects performed in Japan, the scientist demonstrated that the root contained pfaffic acid which he says is capable of inhibiting certain types of cancerous cells. The root, processed and applied to people

□

with cancer, showed "positive" results, Takemoto reports. In addition, the researchers wrote that pfaffia paniculata posesses therapeutical properties that combat anemia, bronchitis, cholesterol, diabetes, fatigue and tuberculosis, among other infirmities.

It is now understood that six saponins called pfaffosides A, B, C, D, E and F are the unique chemicals present in suma which some researchers believe inhibit tumor cell growth. These chemicals are relatively new to science and are said to be found in only one suma, pfaffia paniculata (Martius) Kuntze.

These Japanese studies confirm and reinforce the work being done with suma in Brazil by Dr. Milton Brazzach, Chairman of Pharmacology at the University of Sao Paolo. Dr. Brazzach is said to have been convinced of the power of suma after seeing its results in the treatment of patients, and he now oversees the harvesting of the wild roots of suma.

The suma plant, in addition to saponins, also contains: germanium, a natural metal under analysis for anti-cancer activity; beta-ecdyasone, a substance which may increase the flow of oxygen to cells; allantoin, known to promote wound healing; vitamins, minerals and amino acids; and sitosterol and stigmasterol, plant hormones helpful to human metabolism which are noted for decreasing high blood cholesterol levels and increasing coronary circulation. Sitosterol has also been shown to safely increase the body's natural estrogen, but cannot trigger an excess. This makes suma safe for older women who wish to insure balance and completely banish menopause symptoms, and also avoid the risks of synthetic estrogen replacement therapy, or who also want to avoid "male" tonics such as ginseng, suma proponents state.

This makes suma safe for older women who wish to insure balance and completely banish menopause symptoms . . .

Adapting Properties

The property of acting "only as needed" is characteristic of the whole plant, suma. Like other adaptogens, suma is said to help one to "adapt" to find a new healthy balance. Reactions are not forced, but rather triggered into effect as needed. Put another way, suma simply strengthens the body to a point of higher resistance. In this way, the body's natural immune system has an improved chance of restoring and maintaining one's health.

Suma is available in limited quantites in the U.S. As with pau d' arco and other medicinal herbs, the specific biological pathways to suma's activity in the human body have yet to be determined.

Some of the medical applications of suma are now being tested in the U.S. Among other projects, a program is being initiated to monitor volunteer patients' response to suma.

When more research results come in, suma may indeed turn out to be, as the Brazilians say, "para todo," meaning "for all things." For now, at least, suma can be hailed as a legitimate herbal adaptogen which has a bright future ahead of it.

Available at health food stores. Follow label instructions.

Turmeric And Curcumin

Mukundan, N.A., Chacko, M.C. et al: Effect of turmeric and curcumin on BP-DNA adducts. *Carcinogenesis* 14:493-6,1993.

Many plant constituents, including turmeric, appear to be antimutagens and antioxidants. The modulatory effect of turmeric and curcumin (the oleoresin of turmeric) on the levels of benzo[a]pyrene induced DNA adducts in livers of rats was studied. Turmeric, when fed at 0.1, 0.5, and 3% and curcumin at 0.03% of the diet for four weeks, significantly reduced the levels of BP-DNA adducts formed within 24 hours following a single intraperitoneal injection of benzo[a]pyrene. The significance in terms of potential anti-carcinogenic effect of turmeric is discussed. The results strengthen the role of turmeric as a dietary anti-cancer agent.

Most of our focus regarding the anti-cancer potential of plants has been on bioflavonoids and their powerful antioxidant activity. It is interesting to note the significant number of studies that are also being published looking at spices and other active constituents of plants as cancer preventive due to their ability to inhibit and modulate the early stages of cancer

The results of the studies strengthen the role of turmeric as a dietary anti-cancer agent.

formation. Common food constituents like turmeric, garlic, and the polypenols (i.e., epigallocatechin) found in green or black tea, have all been shown to prevent cancer formation in animal models. These studies have effectively complemented human epidemiological studies indicating the role these foods and spices have played in cancer prevention.

The above study, performed in India, indicates that human intake of turmeric at levels of 0.1-0.5% of the diet present an anti-cancer potential. This equals approximately 500 mg. in a 50 kg. individual. Estimates of turmeric intake in India range from 200 to 600 mg. daily. Incorporating higher intake of turmeric along with garlic, green tea and other food sources of flavonoids may prove the answer in the prevention and reduction of several cancers.

Spicy Yellow Root for Pinkeye?

An Indian pharmaceutical firm is marketing eyedrops made from the common spice turmeric root (curcuma longa). Turmeric, known as Haridra in the Ayurvedic medical tradition of India, has been used for millennia. The efficacy of the Haridras Eyedrops in cases of conjunctivitis (pinkeye) was studied by C. Srinivas and K.V.S. Prabhakaran of the Dept. of Ophthalmology, Government Nizamia General Hospital and Ayurvedic College, Hyderbad, India.

The researchers reported 50 cases treated with Haridras Eyedrops compared to Soframycine Eyedrops, a leading antibiotic. The results indicate that the Haridras drops have a definite role in dealing with conjunctivitis, especially against the bacteria E. Coli, Staph. aureus, Klebsella, and Pseudomonas. The study was reported in *Ancient Science of Life* (April '89).

The eyedrops are prepared pharmaceutically from curcumin, a compound isolated from turmeric root. The authors conclude that turmeric drops are an inexpensive, harmless, and easily available treatment, especially for developing countries. The researchers have previously published research on licorice root (glycyrrhiza glabra) as a promising remedy for eye diseases. *Bepha Bulletin*, Oct.'89.

Eyedrops made from turmeric have a definite role in dealing with conjunctivitis, especially against the bacteria E. Coli, Staph. aureus, Klebsella, and Pseudomonas.

Chapter 9

More Herbal Alternatives To Prescription Medicines

Cayenne And Cluster Headaches

Cluster headaches are more painful than migraines, affecting men more than women. The attacks last 30 to 45 minutes, can occur several times per day and last for weeks or months. At an International Headache Congress in Washington, D.C. (July, 1991), 1,000 headache researchers from 43 countries heard about some of the latest research, including pressurized oxygen, bright lights, and cayenne extract.

The active ingredient in cayenne or red pepper (capsicum spp.) is an oil-based compound called capsaicin. This chemical has made news recently as a new topical application for shingles caused by the herpes zoster virus. Now one study indicates that cluster headache sufferers got significant relief when a capsaicin solution was applied to the nostrils on the same side of the head as the headache. There was no relief when the capsaicin was applied to the other nostril only. Capsaicin apparently works by depleting "Substance P," a pain transmitter in the central nervous system.

One of the presentations at the conference noted that the temples of headache sufferers indicate a heat loss during cluster attacks. Simply rubbing a capsaicin ointment to the temples helped keep sufferers headache-free on days when they would normally experience pain and be in agony. Capsaicin has a noted counter-irritant action; i.e., it produces circulation to the skin area. This may account for the increased heat in the temples,

Cluster headache sufferers got significant relief when the solution was applied to the nostrils on the same side of the head as the headache.

and possibly the apparent prophylactic activity against cluster headaches. (Associated Press in the *Austin-American Statesman*, July 4, 1991)

Cure For Hepatitis B?

"If you contract hepatitis B, don't call your doctor, call your travel agent."

Hepatitis B infection has reached epidemic proportions in much of the world, and has become a serious problem in the U.S. as well. Immunization programs have been implemented and urged for nearly all high-risk groups, including health care workers.

This brings into the realm of possibility some scary questions: what will happen to you when doctors become, not a source of cure, but a source of infection? If you do visit your doctor or dentist more than once a year, are you willing to subject yourself to agonizing innoculations before they touch you, as they do before they come in contact with you? If not, you are in terrifying danger of contracting the potentially deadly hepatitis B from their hands, or their instruments, or even their examining chairs and tables.

This potentially fatal liver disease, also referred to as "serum hepatitis," has long been considered to be a permanent infection. Survivors of the acute phase of the disease carry the virus for life and can have recurring bouts of illness when their resistance is reduced. They can also infect others, although, like AIDS, hepatitis B is a blood-borne disease, not easily transmitted by casual contact.

For over 2,000 years, plants of the genus phyllanthus have been used in Indian Ayurvedic medicine to treat liver disease, including jaundice. The plants have also been used in China, the Philippines, Cuba, Nigeria, Guam, East and West Africa, the Caribbbean, and Central and South America. Modern research on the plant has been under way for over a decade.

Hepatitis B infection has reached epidemic proportions in much of the world, and has become a serious problem in the U.S. as well.

This anti-germotic can destroy the hepatitis B virus if it gains entry into your body.

This anti-germotic, phyllanthus amarus, can not only defend you against hepatitis B in doctors' and dentists' offices, it can destroy the virus if it gains entry into your body through any means whatsoever.

Research conducted in India has shown that phyllanthus amarus can effectively eliminate the virus from the body in 59 percent of cases treated. The clinical research, reported in the prestigious British journal *Lancet*, is coauthored by Nobel Laureate B. S. Blumberg, Ph.D. Dr. Blumberg received his Nobel prize for discovery of the hepatitis B virus and development of the blood test used to detect it.

In this clinical trial, 78 patients were selected, all carriers of the virus. Within the group, 28 were symptom-free carriers, while others had active, chronic liver disease. Treatment consisted of 200 mg of dried, powdered phyllanthus herb (the whole plant, minus roots) in capsules, taken three times per day for 30 days. Lactose was used as a placebo. Both treated and placebo groups returned to the clinic for testing and interviews for at least three months, and some had been followed for nine months at the time of publication of the study. By the first follow-up visit, 59 percent of the treated subjects had no detectable antibodies to the virus, indicating there was absolutely no virus left in their body. Only 4 percent of the placebo group had become seronegative for hepatitis B virus. In no case has the antibody returned in any of the patients who were successfully treated with phyllanthus. After follow-up, only one of the placebo-treated subjects remained virus-free. No toxicity or side effects could be attributed to the drug (or the placebo). This is confirmed by absence of toxicity in animal studies which preceded the clinical tests.

As we have noted before, this natural remedy, like others, will likely not be pursued in the U.S. because of the extreme expense of FDA-required drug approval procedures, and the insufficient profitability to drug companies who would need to bear the expense. Frustration with the regulatory barriers to safe and effective plant-derived medications has led one of our physician friends to remark, "If you contract hepatitis B, don't call your doctor, call your travel agent."

Huckleberries And Cataracts

Huckleberries (also called bilberries, whortleberries or hurtleberries) contain flavonoid-like compounds called anthocyanosides. These compounds have strong antioxidant properties. Some research indicates they may be an even stronger antioxidant than vitamin E (*Et. Radicauz Lubres* 1985).

Extracts of bilberry (vaccinium myrtillus), in combination with vitamin E, have now been used successfully to stop the progression of senile cortical cataracts.

In one recent study, cataract development was stopped cold in 97 percent of the 50 patients involved (*Ann Ottalmol Clin Ocul* 89;115:109). Depending on the products used and the patient, necessary dosages can vary somewhat. Generally, between 25 and 40 drops of bilberry extract, twice daily, and from 400 IU to 800 IU of vitamin E have been the recommended dosages.

Bilberry extracts are not, as yet, very abundant in this country. Bilberry is known mostly for its flavonoid activity which makes varicose veins shrink overnight and bruises disappear. In Russia, the berries have been used as a diuretic for centuries and, with them, gastric colitis, irritable bowel syndrome and other stomach conditions fade away to normalcy in a matter of weeks.

Nettles Tested Against Hay Fever

A study conducted at the National College of Naturopathic Medicine tested the effects of freeze-dried nettles (urtica dioica) on 98 hay fever sufferers. Sixty-nine of the patients finished the trial, which involved subjective evaluation of symptomatic relief using a questionnaire. According to

In one recent study, cataract development was stopped cold in 97 percent of the 50 patients involved.

> **50 percent indicated they would throw away their prescription hay fever medications and use this natural healer instead.**

the evaluation of the patients, 57 percent in the test group judged the urtica to be moderately or highly effective. Half of these patients found it to be "as effective" or "more effective" than previous hay fever medications and the same 50 percent indicated that they would throw away their prescription hay fever medications and purchase and use this natural healer instead. By comparison, 35 percent in the placebo group found the placebo moderately or highly effective but 85 percent of the placebo group considered it less effective than previous hay fever medications and indicated that they would not buy it. According to the study's author, Paul Mittman, "urtica dioica was rated higher than placebo in the global assessment. Comparing the diary data, urtica dioica was rated only slightly higher." ("Randomized, Double-Blind Study of Freeze-Dried Urtica dioica in the Treatment of Allergic Rhinitis" *Planta Medica*. 1990, 56, pgs 44-46).

Tea Tree And Trichomonas

One of the new uses for Tea Tree oil is against trichomonas vaginitis.

Although tea tree oil is available in health food stores and can be used without the guidance of a health professional, the treatment for trichomonas is comparatively complicated and should be used along with visits to your physician.

Trichomonas infections of the vagina are increasingly common and the current medical treatment is considered undesirable because of the many side effects. The most frequently employed compound is called Flagyl (metronidazole). It is carcinogenic, and often produces signs of liver toxicity, nervous system disorder, fatigue, and reduced white blood cell count. Severe reactions may occur if alcohol is consumed during the 10-14 day treatment with Flagyl.

Dr. Eduardo Pena, in Miami, Florida, conducted an extensive clinical evaluation of tea tree oil on 130 cases of vaginal and cervical infections, including 116 that that were diagnosed trichomonal. Once per week, during an office visit and checkup on the progress of treatment, each patient received topical application of tea tree oil and a saturated tampon made of three small sponges that was to be retained for up to 24 hours. The women then used daily douches with tea tree oil between office visits.

Average treatment time was six weeks, and during that time none of the patients reported irritation, burning, or other type of adverse reaction to the treatment. Furthermore, the patients were favorably impressed with the oil's fragrance and its cooling, soothing effect. As controls, he treated 50 cases of trichomonas vaginitis with standard pharmaceutical treatments, using suppositories rather than oral medication. Results with the pharmaceutical agents were no better than those with tea tree oil. In other words, it is already as powerful as the strongest antibiotics for vaginal infections, but the antibiotics will become powerless overnight while this anti-germotic natural oil will go on slaughtering these bacteria forever.

Tea tree oil is often sold as 40 percent emulsion in water with a small amount of alcohol. For use as a douche, a 0.4 percent concentration is adequate, which means that only about one-third fluid ounce of the commercial oil is added to a quart of water, even though larger amounts can be used without harm. For the topical applications and the saturated tampons, Dr. Pena found that higher concentrations are necessary, up to 20 percent (that is, diluting the commercial oil with an equal amount of water).

The action of tea tree oil is largely attributed to its camphor-like terpenes which have the unique action of mixing with sebaceous secretions and thus entering under the top layers of skin. In this way, the disinfecting action is brought to deep level.

Tea tree oil has also been clinically tested in the treatment of furnucles (boils) by Dr. Henry Feinblatt in New York City. In 25 patients with boils, the tea tree oil was applied full strength (that is, the 40 percent dilution commonly available). In 60 percent of the cases the boil disappeared completely, without incisions, within just 8 days, while in another 24 percent

Furthermore, the antibiotics will become powerless overnight while this anti-germotic natural oil will go on slaughtering these bacteria forever.

Where infected wounds had resisted other treatments even for several months, tea tree oil cleared up the condition within one week.

of the cases it had been reduced by more than half in the 8 days. Only one person required incision to drain the infected site. In contrast, an untreated control group of ten patients showed no persons healed within eight days, and 50 percent of the group required incision.

This work was predated by a 1930 report in the *Medical Journal of Australia* which said that a 10 percent solution of tea tree oil could be applied to infected and unclean wounds and that it would dissolve pus, carry out dead cells, and clear away imbedded dirt, leaving the tissues of natural color and free of infection. In cases where infected wounds had resisted other treatments even for several months, the use of tea tree oil cleared up the condition within one week.

Chapter 10

Cancer Treatment On Your Grocery Shelf?

B ENZALDEHYDE IS A CHEMICAL found in nature in many foods. It helps give coffee and cocoa their pleasant aromas and is widely used in the chemical industry.

Less known is the fact that benzaldehyde has shown significant cancer-fighting abilities. In the early 1970's, Japanese scientists used a distillate of figs to successfully treat cancer in mice. They eventually found that the active ingredient which had the cancer-killing power was ordinary benzaldehyde, present in mere one-part-per-million concentrations.

In 1985, Dr. M. Kochi and colleagues reported in the U.S. National Cancer Institute's own *Cancer Treatment Reports* (69:533-7) that a gluconated form of benzaldehyde called (BG) caused an overall response of 55 percent. Seven patients (11 percent) achieved complete remission, 29 (45 percent) achieved partial response, 24 (37 percent) showed no more progress of the disease and 5 (8 percent) showed progressive disease.

A 1990 report by Dr. Tatsumura and colleagues at Toyama University confirmed similar responses.

And, in all cases, the treatment was free of toxicity.

It is thus documented, safe, inexpensive — and generally not available in America.

How is it possible that such a promising anti-cancer agent is unused here? Why hasn't the NCI publicized these results as they have the taxol trials?

Benzaldehyde, found in ordinary almond extract, has shown significant cancer-fighting abilities. In all cases, the treatment was free of toxicity.

One reason is that pharmaceutical companies have little incentive to become involved in research on natural food constituents. It currently costs over $230 million to shepherd a new drug through the FDA's approval maze.

Benzaldehyde is too cheap. About 30 cents an ounce at chemical supply houses. Such companies do sell benzaldehyde but you have to sign a pledge that it's not to be used for medicine. Since the average person needs less than a gram a day, the cost per year would be about $2.00.

Pharma-ceutical companies have little incentive to become involved in research on natural food constituents. Benzaldehyde is too cheap, about 30 cents an ounce.

Benzaldehyde is still investigative, so please don't abandon other treatments to take it. However, your health professional might be interested in supplementing your current program with it.

An odd but easy way to get a measurable dose of benzaldehyde is from the ordinary almond extract found in supermarkets — either pure or artificial. Both contain between 2.0 and 2.5 percent benzaldehyde. About 700 milligrams in each ounce.

How much is a therapeutic dose?

Can't tell for sure, but extrapolating from the Japanese experiments, a 150 pound person could use around 560 milligrams. Or, ¾ of an ounce of almond extract in a glass of fruit juice divided into four equal doses for a day.

Benzaldehyde is generally regarded as safe (GRAS) by the FDA. However, at high doses it can be dangerous. Between 1.7 and 2.0 ounces of pure benzaldehyde can be fatal. That translates into about 50 bottles of almond extract ingested at one time.

Some doctors are open to the prospect of treatment options, while other are not.

Chapter 11

Chronic Fatigue Syndrome And Malic Acid

CHRONIC FATIGUE? And Your Doctor Has No Answers . . . Fibromyalgia is another one of those "catch all" con ditions that refers to pain and inflammation of muscles, tendons, ligaments and the connective tissue around joints. Now we've learned that the same supplements that help fibromyalgia are often effective in treating chronic fatigue syndrome.

Doctors have reported that malic acid is a safe, inexpensive treatment that wipes out chronic fatigue syndrome in about 49 percent of those treated so far (*Health Watch* 93;3(1):1,3).

Malic acid is a natural substance extracted from apples. In the body, along with magnesium, it is one of the components in the energy-producing Krebs cycle in which fats and sugar are converted to pure energy.

The products available usually contain 300 milligrams of magnesium hydroxide in addition to malic acid. At this strength, the recommended dosage has generally been between 6 and 12 tablets daily taken with food and water. While patients suffering from fibromyalgia often see an improvement within 48 hours, those suffering from chronic fatigue syndrome may need to take the supplement for at least two weeks before seeing improvement. Once the desired effect is achieved the dosage can be tapered off over time.

If you can't find malic acid in your health food store, try the C.F.I.D.S. Buyers Club, 1187 Coast Village Road, Suite #1-280, Santa Barbara, CA 93108, or call 1-800-366-6056.

Malic acid is a safe, inexpensive treatment that wipes out chronic fatigue syndrome in about 49 percent of those treated.

Chapter 12

More Than "Fun" In Fungi

Mushrooms like the shiitake, reishi, and maitake can have astoundingly beneficial effects on health.

PLANTS CREATE FOOD by means of the action of chlorophyll and sunlight, carbon dioxide and water.

Fungi cannot do this.

They have no chlorophyll and cannot produce their own food. Instead, they live on other living, dead or decaying things.

Sounds ghoulish!

However, mushrooms are fungi and some mushrooms like the shiitake, reishi, and maitake can have astoundingly beneficial effects on health and can contribute to the cure of such serious illnesses as influenza, neuralgia, high blood pressure, and cancer.

Mushrooms have been cultivated as a food for thousands of years. In the Orient, shiitake mushrooms are cultivated as both a food and a medicine. They can be added to your diet in four ways. They can be eaten raw in salads when they are fresh, or if dried when you buy them, eaten after you soak them in twice their weight in water for twenty minutes. Don't discard any leftover water. You can brew a tea with chopped shiitake mushrooms or you can make a very strong extract by heating powdered shiitake in enough water to cover over a low heat until half the water has been evaporated. Strain while still hot.

Of course, you can buy tablets which contain the concentrated extract of the shiitake mushroom at your health food store.

Brewed shiitake tea and shiitake extract are almost always used in curing disease. An average daily dose of shiitake tea consists of two dried mushrooms steeped in about one cup of hot water, but the dose or the number of tablets to be taken depends on the nature of the sickness being treated. The substances found in shiitake are able to contribute to the cure of virus-caused disease in a number of ways. They stimulate your body to make antibodies against the attacking organism. Also, the shiitake is said to contain components which stimulate the manufacture of interferon which establishes a protective barrier against the spread of the virus in your body. For a day or two, the super-viruses may penetrate into your body. But they can't spread there, and if they can't spread, they can't infect you, and they die. And then they're flushed out like the garbage they are.

The immune booster found in shiitake is called lentinan (technically, it's a polysaccharide). Japanese scientists have concluded that lentinan should be effective for the patient with advanced or recurrent stomach or colorectal cancer in combination with chemotherapeutic agents.

Lentinan is approved for this use by the Japanese regulatory authorities. Do viruses cause cancers? No, they trigger them. They start them growing inside your body — unless you slash off those triggers with these anti-germotics. Lentinan, for example, prevents chemicals and viruses from triggering cancer and is considered one of the most effective agents for controlling small metastases. (Taguchi, T. "Effects of lentinan in advanced or recurrent cases of gastric, colorectal, and breast cancer." *Gan To Kagaku Ryoho*, 1983; 10:387-93.)

Scientists Rose, W.C. et al. reported in *Cancer Research*, "Immunotherapy of Madison 109 lung carcinoma and other tumors using lentinan," 1984;44:1368-73., that even if lentinan therapy was begun after tumors had enlarged, the results were astounding. In-depth examination showed no tumors left and a complete cure of up to 63 percent of laboratory mice in three separate experiments.

For a day or two, the super-viruses may penetrate into your body. But they can't spread there and infect you. They die and then they're flushed out like the garbage they are.

The lentinan used in these tests was a purified extract produced and patented by Ajinmoto, the huge Japanese chemical company, but not approved for use in the United States.

However, shiitake mushrooms are available in the United States and, although more expensive than the traditional mushrooms you find in most markets, can be used therapeutically as well as gastronomically.

Lentinan As A Model For The Efficacy Of Immunomodulators In Cancer And HIV-Infection

Do viruses cause cancers? No, they trigger them — unless you slash off those triggers with these anti-germotics.

Chihara, G. "Recent progress in immunopharmacology and therapeutic effects of polysaccharides" *Develop Biol Standard* 77:191-7, 1992.

Lentinan (from lentinus edodes, shiitake mushroom), has been shown to have marked antitumor activity to suppress chemical and viral oncogenesis and prevent cancer recurrence or metastasis ofter surgery. Results of the clinical application of lentinan have shown prolongation of life span of patients with advanced and recurrent stomach, colorectal and breast cancer with minimal side effects. These polysaccharides also increase host resistance to various bacterial, viral and parasitic infections. Lentinan is presented as an example of a Host Defense Potentiator (HDP), which can restore or augment the ability of responsiveness of the host to lymphocytokines or other intrinsic bioactive factors through maturation, differentiation or proliferation of the critical cells for host defense mechanisms. HDP's appear to make the physiological constitution highly cancer and infection and disease-proof — a concept in Oriental Medicine which deals with the regulation of the homeostasis of the whole body, thus bringing a diseased person to a more balanced or normal state (i.e., adaptogen). HDP's like lentinan are the most appropriate drugs to prevent cancer recurrence, or the manifestation of AIDS symptoms in those infected with HIV.

Shiitake is not the only naturally protective member of the mushroom family. Enter mushroom number two, the reishi (ganoderma), also known as the longevity herb of the Orient.

Reishi (Ganoderma lucidum and G. applanatum) have traditionally been used against cancer for hundreds of years. Polysaccharides derived from the mushroom are patented in Japan for use as immunomodulators in cancer treatments. They are usually combined with chemo and radio-therapies to reduce side effects, increase the efficacy of the treatment, and to accelerate recovery from disease. They have been combined with large doses of vitamin C, (6-12 grams a day) as a mixture of ascorbic acid and sodium ascorbate, to increase their activity.

The original textbook of Oriental medical science, *Shinnoh Honsohkyo*, classified and explained the uses of 365 medicines. Medicines were divided into three classes: Superior medicines, sometimes called, "God's Herbs," which were used to perpetuate youth and promote longevity and were part of the magician's arsenal. Average Medicines were used as tonics. Fair Medicines had to be monitored and not taken on a daily basis. The Superior Medicines could be taken 365 days a year.

One of the leading Superior Medicines in the text was the reishi.

Reishi is a basidomycete, a mushroom of the Polyporaceae family. There are more than 2,000 kinds of mushrooms in this family, each with a distinct shape and form and most of them with protective ability if eaten or, as in China, used by injection, as a tincture, syrup or in tablet form.

Alexander Solzhenitsyn, in his novel *The Cancer Ward*, mentions a mushroom that lives on white birch trees. He called them tchaga and notes that farmers have been eating them for centuries and escaping cancer without even being aware of it. The tchaga is botanically known as betula taus-chii.

The idea that mushrooms may be healing is foreign to the average American. The closest the American has come to recognizing mushroom power was when the "magic mushroom" of hallucinogenic fame was

Reishi mushrooms have traditionally been used against cancer for hundreds of years.

This is a powerful admission by the goverment that certain foods play an important part in disease prevention.

reported in many newspapers and TV shows. So, when the following story appeared in the Japanese newspaper *Hokubei Mainichi* on October 4, 1980, the Japanese public was prepared to accept it as truth . . . while the American press didn't even bother to report it and western medicine scoffed at it:

A virus in Japanese mushrooms can be made to produce interferon, effective in treating cancer and viruses, it has been confirmed in a joint study by the medical department of Kobe University and the Nippon Kinoko Institute. According to professor Manabu-Takeharu, spherical particles of virus under the caps contain double-stranded DNA, effective not only in restraining intrusion into the cells, but also capable of inducing cells to manufacture interferon. It's the tamed virus that makes you virus-proof.

We ignored this information.

The Japanese purified the material, concentrated it, standardized it and made it into tablets and a healing miracle.

In Oriental medicine there is a term called "Mi-Byo" which translates into "presumptive disease." It is an important concept because a person in Mi-Byo will become sick if the condition is not treated. The condition of Mi-Byo is neither health nor illness, but a presumptive sick condition.

With the modern conditions that assail us today — stress, pollution, free radicals, environmental insults — many of us are Mi-Byo. Recently, there has been a spate of information about adding cruciferous vegetables to our diet to help ward off disease. This is a powerful admission by the goverment that certain foods play an important part in disease prevention. This is precisely what the ancient Orientals were saying when they granted Superior Medicine status to the reishi, except they didn't have the clinical evidence at that time. Since the reishi functions as a stimulant to health, including the prevention or improvement of degenerative diseases without fear of side effects with long usage, it is ideal for Mi-Byo.

Anti-Inflammatory Reishi

In a paper presented at the Third Academic/Industry Joint Conference in Sapporo, Japan, in 1990, pharmacologist William Stavinoha (University of Texas Health Science Center, San Antonio) elucidated his investigations into Ganoderma lucidum. This mushroom, the reishi mushroom, was classified over 2,000 years ago as a superior medicine. Using two pharmacologic tests, Dr. Stavinoha showed Ganoderma exhibits strong anti-inflammatory activity with "no untoward effects." In this experiment, the Ganoderma extracts were compared to the well-known anti-inflammatory agents hydrocortisone, phenylbutazone, and aspirin, all of which have serious side effects and toxicity. The activity of the gill powder (spores) from Ganoderma mushrooms gave as much relief from inflammation as hydrocortisone and aspirin, and exceeded the activity of phenylbutazone, but with none of their deadly side effects. The spores were effective both orally and as topical applications. (Stavinoha, W. (Aug. 1990) Third Academic/Industry Joint Conference in Sapporo, Japan. Unpublished.)

Chihara, G: Recent progress in immunopharmacology and therapeutic effects of polysaccharides. *Develop Biol Standard* 77: 191-7, 1992.

Lentinan (from lentinus edode [shiitake mushroom]) has been shown to have marked antitumor activity, suppress chemical and viral pro-cancerous effects, and prevent cancer recurrence or metastasis after surgery. Results of the clinical application of lentinan have shown prolongation of life span of patients with advanced and recurrent stomach, colorectal and breast cancer with minimal side effects. These polysaccharides also increase host resistance to various bacterial, viral, and parasitic infections. Lentinan is presented as an example of a Host Defense Potentiator (HDP), which can augment and strengthen the response of the immunoreactive cells. HDP's appear to make the physiological constitution highly cancer and infection-resistant — a concept in Oriental Medicine which deals with the regulation of the homeostasis of the whole body, thus bringing a dis-

The mushrooms gave as much relief from inflammation as hydro-cortisone and aspirin, but with none of their deadly side effects.

eased person to a more balanced or normal state (i.e., adaptogen). HDP's like lentinan are the most appropriate drugs to prevent cancer recurrence, or to slow manifestation of AIDS symptoms in those infected with HIV.

The vast potential for immunomodulators of plant origin in the long-term management of cancer and HIV-infected patients continues to be largely ignored in this country. Research in Japan, Europe, and Africa continues to point to the improvement in quality of life when incorporating plant medicines that have previously been described as tonics or adaptogens. Plants meeting this criteria include astragalus, eleutherococcus (siberian ginseng), shisandra, and shiitake mushroom.

A common characteristic of these phytomedicines is the presence of high amounts of complex polysaccharides. Many of them also contain complex glycosides that are not only immunomodulating but also have a supportive effect on adrenal function — a critical consideration in any chronic illness.

Maitake Mushrooms

Now that you've become comfortable and conversant with shiitake and reishi mushrooms and the fact that they are available at health food stores, we will introduce you to the "king" of the mushrooms . . . Maitake!

Welcome the maitake (grifola frondosa), also known as the "Dancing Mushroom." The name comes either from dancing with joy when it is found or from the way the fruit bodies overlap each other, giving the appearance of butterflies dancing in the wind.

Maitake is a big mushroom (almost the size of a basketball) found in the northeastern mountains of Japan. For many years, the local natives prized this rare and tasty mushroom for its health benefits. Until now, it could not be cultivated, but recently a method was developed and it is now available in the United States. Based on recent studies, the maitake mush-

Now, we will introduce you to the "king" of mushrooms. For many years, the local natives prized this rare and tasty mushroom for its health benefits.

room is known as the most potent immunostimulant among all the mushrooms and other polysaccharide compounds.

As have all the other mushrooms and herbs described in this book, maitake has been called an adaptogen, the term used to describe the multiple effects these substances have on the body. Adaptogens are defined as substances having a balancing effect on the body irrespective of the particular illness.

A common denominator among mushroom and herbal adaptogens is the presence of complex polysaccharides, long chains of sugar molecules with a known protective effect on human health, particularly the immune system. These active components, whether virus, polysaccharide or other, have the unique ability to act as immunomodulators and have thus become a central focus of cancer and AIDS research. The polysaccharide found in maitake has a unique structure said to be the most powerful investigated to date. So maitake is being investigated as a potential tool in the management of numerous destructive ailments, including cancer, diabetes, hypertension, obesity, and HIV-infection.

So far, the most extensive area of research has been in the area of anti-cancer activity. Maitake has been shown over and over again to stop the growth of breast cancer cells, lung cancer cells and skin cancer cells in experiments done on laboratory mice.

(Proc. Intl. Symp. Scientific and Technical Aspects of Cultivating Fungus, Penn. State Univ., 1986, pp. 1-6.)

Orally adminstered maitake mushroom powder was able to stop tumor growth in 86 of 100 mice, with 4 out 10 animals completely cured.

In Japan, maitake extract is currently being studied against leukemia, prostate cancer, uterine cancer, ovarian cancer, and fibroid tumors, but the ramifications extend beyond just cancer. New research appears to show that maitake has the ability to prevent HIV from killing T-lymphocytes. The death of the T-lymphocytes is a critical factor in the progression of an HIV-infected individual to AIDS.

Maitake has been shown over and over again to stop the growth of breast cancer cells, lung cancer cells, and skin cancer cells.

Their own documents show that maitake inhibited the growth of the HIV virus at about the same rate as the toxic drug AZT.

At a conference held at Kyushu Industrial College in Fukuoka, Japan, on March 29, 1992, Dr. Hiroaki Nanba announced that a maitake extract was able to prevent HIV destruction of T-lymphocytes by as much as 96 percent in vitro.

If you can find maitake msuhrooms in your local food store, eat them for health and for their considerable culinary delight. A more concentrated dosage of the whole fruiting body of high quality maitake is now available in tablet form and is highly recommended. Vitamin C has been shown to increase the bioavailability of complex polysaccharides so it's worth taking along with your maitake tablet.

What about research in the United States?

Is there some sort of plot to prevent possible treatments from being used?

The National Cancer Institute was shown results of maitake tests in 1991. Their own documents show that, in their tests, maitake inhibited the growth of the HIV virus at about the same rate as the toxic drug AZT. For reasons of its own, however, NCI chose to first "sulfate" maitake extract, thus rendering it toxic!

Who said that?

None other than Ralph W. Moss, Ph.D., in his book, *Cancer Therapy*, Equinox Press, New York 1992. Dr. Moss was assistant director of public affairs at Memorial Sloan-Kettering Cancer Center.

Maitake Mushroom — Antitumor Activity And Clinical Update

Hishida, I., Nanba, H. and Kuoda, H: Antitumor activity exhibited by orally administered extract from fruit body of Grifolia frondosa (Maitake). *Chem Pharm Bull* 36:1819-27, 1988.

A polysaccharide, 3-branched beta 1,6 glucan, extracted from the fruit bodies of grifolia frondosa (maitake mushroom) exhibited antitumor activites against allogenic and sygeneic tumors on oral administration to mice. Winn assay conducted to examine the tumor growth-suppressing effect revealed a complete inhibition of the tumor by administration of the polysaccharide. Examination of the effect of this polysaccharide extract on immune response indicated enhancement of the cytolytic activity and interleukin-1 productivity of macrophages and T cells. It was also shown to potentiate the delayed-type hypersensitivity response which is associated with tumor growth suppression.

The last ten years have seen the influx of several "medicinal mushrooms" including shiitake and reishi. This influx is a result of extensive research indicating immunomuodulating and antitumor activites of polysaccharides extracted from these mushrooms. Maitake mushroom, also known as the "Dancing mushroom," has been used for years in various Japanese recipes and also as a tonic or adaptogen. Clinical research with maitake has increased dramatically in the past six years with a great deal of the focus centering on the anti-tumor activity of its unique polysaccharide component (shiitake has a 6-branched beta 1,3 glucan polysaccharide). Research in Japan has presented maitake as a potential tool in the management of cancer, HIV-infection, diabetes, hpertension, hypercholesterolemia, and obesity.

Getting back to anti-tumor potential, the unique aspect of the maitake polysaccharide is its ability to be effectively utilized when taken orally (Yamada, Y., Nanba, H. & Kuroda, H.: *Chemotherapy* 38:790-6, 1990). Most studies have demonstrated that other polysaccharide extracts from mushroom sources (i.e., lentinan from shiitake) must be administered intravenously to have effect. In a head-to-head study with shiitake in rats with experimentally-induced tumors, maitake demonstrated superior ability to inhibit tumor growth (Mori, K. et al: *Proc Intl Symp Scientific and Technical Aspects of Cultivating Fungus* Penn State Univ., 1986, pp 1-6). Using an allogenic tumor model (Sarcoma 180), maitake demonstrated an 86.3 percent inhibition of tumor growth thirty-one days after implantation versus 77.9 percent for shiitake (powdered concentrates of the fruiting body was

Clinical research with maitake has increased dramatically in the past six years.

Four of the ten mice in the maitake group had complete tumor resolution and this has led to human clinical trials.

added to the animals' feed). Four of the ten mice in the maitake group had complete tumor resolution. This research has led to human clinical trials in Japan with leukemia, prostate cancer, uterine cancer, ovarian cancer, and fibroid tumors.

Maitake has also been in the news with regard to HIV-infection. At the conference held at Kyushu Industrial College, Dr. Hiroaki Nanbe also announced that the previously mentioned polysaccharide in a sulfated form was able to inhibit HIV-destruction of CD4 cells by as much as 97 percent. Preliminary reports on the anti-HIV activity of the sulfated polysaccharide from maitake have also been issued by both the Japanese National Institutes of Health as well as the National Cancer Institute in the U.S. These preliminary results obviously do not confirm this activity in humans, but do point toward the initiation of clinical trials in the near future.

The concentrate of the whole fruiting body of maitake that is currently available in this country is being examined clinically by a number of physicians on the East coast. It is important to point out that in the case of maitake, the fruit body is higher in polysaccharides than the mycelium stage (immature stage between the spore and mature fruit body) which is used in many reishi and shiitake extracts. Hopefully, a more concentrated extract with standardized polysaccharide content will soon be available to physicians in the U.S.

Anti-HIV Activity Found In Maitake Mushroom

Maitake has been recognized for its wide medicinal properties for high blood pressure and diabetes as well. Voluntary-base trial programs have been underway in U.S.A. with people with AIDS and cancer patients and such medicinal effects are being confirmed there.

The group has studied polysaccharides, named glucan, extracted from the maitake. Through the tests, by adding a chemical compound of the glucan to HIV infected Helper T-cells in vitro, it confirmed the inhibition of HIV activities.

Once infected by HIV, Helper T-cells are eventually destroyed. Prof. Nanba claimed in his report, however, that such HIV activity has been inhibited by the chemical compound of maitake glucan. In the in vitro test, 97 percent of the 300,000 HIV infected T-cells remained alive with the minimal amount of 1/100,000 gram of maitake compound.

Concerning anti-cancer activites, it has been confirmed that the glucan enhances the immune-related cells' activities, such as macrophages and natural killer cells which fight against cancers. In the animal test, tumors of about one-half of mice completely disappeared and those of the other half were significantly diminished.

Further, it is also confirmed that a substance extracted from maitake (other than glucan) demonstrates activities of lowering the sugar content level in your blood as well as lowering your blood pressure. Ms. Keiko Okubo, a researcher of the group, has made a detailed report on such activities on March 30, 1992 at the same conference in Fukuoka, Japan.

One of the outstanding characteristics of the maitake mushroom is that the extract is effective even in oral administration, unlike other polysaccharides. Studies on antitumor and anti-HIV activities of maitake extract have been also conducted in U.S.A. at the National Cancer Institute of the National Institutes of Health since November 1991, and the results supporting Prof. Nanba's announcement have been reported.

A substance extracted from maitake demonstrates activities of lowering the sugar content level in your blood as well as lowering your blood pressure.

Abstract

The following abstract on Maitake Mushroom has been submitted to VIII International Conference on AIDS/III STD World Congress, 1992;

Significant activation of immune response system may contribute strongly to the inhibition of various diseases caused by secondary infections among HIV carriers.

Title

Immunostimulant Activity (in vivo) and Anti-HIV activity (in vitro) of 3 Branched B-1.6 Glucan Extracted from MAITAKE MUSHROOM

Author

Hiroaki Nanba, Prof., Kobe Women's College of Pharmacy

Objectives

1) Maitake extract, MT-2, was believed to have in vivo immune stimulating activity both by injection and oral administration which is unique to MT-2.
2) Sulfated MT-2 was believed to show potent anti-HIV activity in vitro.

Methods

1) Enhancement of cellular immune system has been examined using tumor-bearing mice with CH3 mice as control. Differences of immune activities between MT-2 treated and non-treated cells were observed.
2) Anti-HIV activities were examined on sulfated MT-2 by microplate method (as widely used at both US and Japan NIH).

Results

1) Activities of machrophage, killer-cells and cyto-toxic T-cells were significantly increased by 1.4, 1.86, and 1.6 times respectively compared to those of non MT-2 treated tumor-bearing mice, which results in 86 percent tumor growth inhibition in tumor-bearing host. (Similiar results were obtained by oral administration of dried powder of MAITAKE MUSHROOM).
2) Microplate tests of sulfated MT-2 demonstrated potent anti-HIV activities in vitro.

Conclusion

Significant immune stimulating activity of MT-2 was confirmed even with oral administration. Anti-tumor activity in vivo as well as anti-HIV activity in vitro were confirmed. It is suggested significant activation of immune response system by MT-2 may contribute strongly to the inhibition of various diseases caused by secondary infections among HIV carriers.

Chapter 13

To Bee

THIS PORTION OF THE BOOK was inspired by this piece of information about bee propolis and colon cancer.

Sweet Route To Heading Off Colon Cancer

In recent years, a host of studies have identified a broad spectrum of medical attributes in honey — including antifungal, antibacterial, anti-inflammatory, antiproliferative, and cancer-drug-potentiating properties. Now, researchers at the American Health Foundation in Valhalla, N.Y., have uncovered another. In *Cancer Research*, Bandaru S. Reddy and his co-workers describe the ability of honey-derived caffeic esters to inhibit the development of precancerous changes in the colon of rats given a known carcinogen.

These esters come from the propolis — the brown, resinous, tree-derived material that honeybees use to cement together their hives. Reddy's group considers three derivatives of the caffeic esters promising enough to use in longer-term animal studies of colon cancer.

So, we followed it a bit further and found out some more about it.

In recent years, a host of studies have identified a broad spectrum of medical attributes in honey...

Caffeic Acid And Cancer

Propolis, a honey beehive product, is thought to exhibit a broad spectrum of activities including antibiotic, antiviral, anti-inflammatory and tumor growth inhibition. Some of the observed biological activities may be due to caffeic acid (cinnamic acid) esters that are present in propolis.

In this study, the authors synthesized three caffeic acid esters, namely methyl caffeate, phenylethyl caffeate, and phenylethyl dimethylcaffeate and tested them against DMAB — (a colon and mammary carcinogen) induced mutagenicity.

The effect of these agents on the growth of human colon adenocarcinoma, HT-29 cells and activities of ornithine decarboxylase and protein tyrosine kinase was also studied. The results indicate that mutagenicity was significantly inhibited with 150 uM methyl caffeate, 40-60 uM of phenylethyl caffeate, and 40-80 uM of phenylethyl dimethylcaffeate. Treatment of HT-29 colon adenocarcinoma cells with these acids significantly inhibited the cell growth and syntheses of RNA, DNA and protein. Ornithine decarboxylase and protein tyrosine kinase activities were also inhibited in HT-29 cells.

These results demonstrate that caffeic acid esters which are present in propolis possess chemopreventive properties when tested in short-term assay systems.

Rao, C. et al. "Effect of caffeic acid esters on carcinogen-induced mutagenicity and human colon adenocarcinoma cell growth." *Chem Biol Interactions*, 1992; 84: 277-290.

Pollen, Honey, Royal Jelly

From propolis we investigated pollen and honey. While honey has been used as a food and medicine since the cave days, the "new" field of natural medicine is leading to another look at all of the products derived from bees and the hive.

In the beginning is Royal Jelly, a pearly-white gelatinous mass produced by the pharyngeal glands located in the heads of the nursing bees. This nectar appears to be one of nature's most concentrated foods. It is rich in

> *Honey has been used as a food and medicine since the cave days. . . This nectar appears to be one of nature's most concentrated foods.*

proteins, trace minerals, B^1, B^2, B^6 and B^{12}. It is a source of niacin, biotin, folic acid and inositol, an excellent source of pantothenic acid, and also contains all of the essential amino acids. Also 10-hydroxy-decenoic acid, now being studied for its anti-cancer activity. It contains acetylcholine, a neurotransmitter needed for proper cell function, and plenty of minerals.

The queen is fed royal jelly all her life and grows to be 40 percent larger and 60 percent heavier than the worker bees, which is incredible since both the queen and the workers come from identical eggs. The only difference is the queen's diet! This high energy food enables the queen bee to lay 2,000 eggs daily — approximately 2 ½ times her total weight.

All due to the daily intake of royal jelly.

For humans, royal jelly is thought to aid mental alertness, provide energy and a general feeling of well-being, aid in cell regeneration, increase resistance to disease and help maintain skin tone and hair health. Furthermore, royal jelly helps trigger an increase in the brain's production of serotonin, an essential for those who have difficulty controlling their appetite, suffer from sleep disorder, or have low energy levels.

If this sounds intriguing, you can get capsules of royal jelly from your health food store.

It was King Solomen who said it best: "Thy lips, O my spouse, drop as the honeycomb: honey and milk are under thy tongue."

Much nicer than the writer who called honey "bee barf." Pliny said it was "a perspiration of the sky or sort of saliva from the stars."

Maybe the bee barf was closer since bees suck nectar from flowers and store it in their honey sacs. Back at the hive, the foraging bees regurgitate nectar into the six-sided honeycombs. Then worker bees take over, ingesting and regurgitating the nectar for about twenty minutes.

Not a pretty picture. But after all, milk is reconstructed cow blood!

Honey is 25 percent sweeter than sugar but has 40 percent more calories: 64 calories to a tablespoon of honey, 46 calories in a tablespoon of sugar. The flavor and aroma of honey is derived from the pollen and nectar

Royal jelly aids mental alertness, provides energy, aids in cell regeneration, and increases resistance to disease.

Mountain climbers at even the highest altitudes have used honey to overcome fatigue and for energy superchargers.

of the supplying flowers. A long time ago, when honey was used for its curative powers, hives were placed near certain grasses, flowers or shrubs. Honey from hives placed in fennel or horehound groves were used for coughs. Hives near foxglove supposedly produced honey to aid heart congestion. Linden honey was used for fever and elderberry and juniper for stomach upsets.

How about honey gathered near marijuana plants? Imagine the consternation of the FDA.

Honey comes to us in its predigested form so it's very easy to digest. Another reason for easy digestion is its high glucose content (also known as blood sugar). One of the important properties of glucose is its ability to restore oxygen to the body by replacing the lactic acid which builds up in fatigued muscle tissues. This explains, in part, why it is preferred as an energy source. Athletes have appreciated it, mountain climbers at even the highest altitudes, and others under physical stress have used honey to overcome fatigue and for energy superchargers. This also makes it an energy miracle for people who are ill or weak.

The spectrum of minerals in honey are in percentages that approximate their concentration in human blood. The darker the honey, the higher the mineral content.

Honey is a natural antiseptic, antibiotic and antimycotic. Honey will not support the growth of bacteria. But, don't ever give it to babies under one year of age !

And, you don't want to eat rhododendron honey.

In 400 B.C., a Greek writer described the side effects of honey gathered from the wrong type of flowers. Those who had eaten a little behaved as though they were drunk, those who had gorged themselves went mad.

Honey from an orange grove is very often labeled orange-blossom honey, but bees gather honey from any flower within their flying range. Raw and unstrained honeys are closest to their natural state and some honey lovers prefer to eat honey and comb together.

Who's Who In The Honeybee's Hive

THE QUEEN: A two-day-old larva picked to be queen gets royal-nursery treatment for 11 days, then emerges from the hive, pursued by about 18 drones. Ten days later, she begins laying eggs, as many as 2,000 per day.

THE DRONES: These stingerless males live only to mate with a queen. Those who succeed drop dead from the sky after their moment of triumph. The lesser studs hang around the hive until food becomes short, then they are booted out.

THE WORKERS: For the other 50,000 to 60,000 females in the hive, life is all work, no play, and usually about 30 days long. A good worker produces one-twelfth of a tablespoon of honey in her lifetime.

More About Bee Propolis — Nature's Antibiotic

More than 30 years ago, researchers discovered that bees, contrary to other insects and animals, were free of any bacteria.

Their hives were "hospital clean."

When you consider that the average hive is smaller than two cubic feet and has a population of 50,000 to 65,000 bees in an environment with a moisture content of 90 percent and a mean temperature of 95 degrees, it should be a perfect breeding ground for bacteria, infection and disease.

But it's not and the answer is propolis.

Propolis, meaning in Greek "defense before a town," is a resinous substance gathered and metabolized by the bees from the bark or leaf buds of deciduous trees. It contains resins, balsam, wax, etheric oils, pollen, vitamins, minerals, amino acids, plus previously discussed caffeic esters and a high level of flavonoids. Bees also use this substance to fill in holes and to make the entrance to the hive small enough to keep out invaders.

More than 30 years ago, researchers discovered that bees, contrary to other insects and animals, were free of any bacteria.

The flavonoids in propolis are about 500 times the potency of oranges and are responsible for its major antibiotic effects.

Intruders who enter the hive are killed and then covered with propolis which mummifies the body. It does not decay and spread disease.

The flavonoids found in propolis are about 500 times the potency and healing power of oranges and are believed to be responsible for the major antibiotic effects of propolis. Flavonoids have numerous therapeutic effects — among them are beneficial actions on the capillary system and the circulatory system, and as a vasodilator. They act as diuretics, increase bile production, and have been reported to influence the production of compounds from the thymus, thyroid, pancreas and adrenal glands.

The ability of propolis to purify makes it effective for healing sore gums or sore throat, and for stomach and intestinal infections.

Propolis is not a "new" discovery. Hippocrates prescribed it to help heal sores and both internal and external ulcers. And in 400 B.C. Herodotus the Greek wrote of propolis ointment to treat open wounds and abscesses.

The Koran and Persian and Arabic manuscripts of the 6th century also mention this substance to treat eczemas, purify the blood and treat bronchial catarrhs.

The Many Roles Of Royal Jelly And Propolis

Among the uses documented in research or history for royal jelly and propolis are the following:

Royal Jelly

- **Antibiotic:** Its bacteria-destroying action helps prevent a diverse range of ailments, from acne and influenza to stomach ulcers and urinary tract infections. Its bioflavonoid content has been found to enhance the effectiveness of Vitamin C in the body.

- **Energy:** Taken as a supplement or in snack products, it helps maintain vigor and stamina.
- **Appetite:** It can help trigger an increase in the production of the brain chemical serotonin, essential for people suffering from appetite control problems, sleep disorders and low energy levels.
- **Immune System:** Its high content of essential nutrients helps boost the immune system.
- **Allergies:** Research has indicated it can aid in controlling allergies.
- **Common Maladies:** It has been found to help relieve constipation, arthritis pain, muscle tension, headache, vertigo and eye fatigue.

Propolis

- **Immune System:** Its high-nutrient profile and antiseptic properties help build resistance to disease.
- **Radiation:** Injuries caused by exposure to radiation have been healed with propolis, according to some research studies. A double-blind test conducted in Yugoslavia revealed improvement in patients treated with propolis for liver problems caused by radiation exposure.
- **Ulcers:** An Austrian physician reported that there was no trace of ulcer pain after three days in 7 out of 10 patients studied and that the wounds in 6 out of 10 patients healed after 10 days.
- **Stamina:** It has been used by many athletes, including world class athletes and Olympic champions, for strength and stamina.
- **Infection:** It has been shown to alleviate sore throats, allergy symptoms, cold sores, acne, ear infections, urinary tract

There was no trace of ulcer pain after three days in 7 out of 10 patients studied.

The flavonoid activity of propolis "may well represent a whole new generation of antibiotic activity."

infections and other infections. Professor Bent Havsteen, formerly of Cornell University and an international expert in the area of propolis, has stated: The flavonoid activity of propolis "may well represent a whole new generation of antibiotic activity." A good deal of this action is attributed to its high bioflavonoid content.

What about Pollen?

Carlson Wade, in his book *ABOUT POLLEN* states: Bee pollen contains a gonadotrophic hormone similar to the pituitary hormone, gonadotrophin, which functions as a sex gland stimulant. (That's enough to make you consider getting a few stings as you raid the bee's pollen bank.)

The healing, rejuvenating, and disease-fighting effects of this total nutrient are hard to believe, yet are fully documented. Aging, digestive upsets, prostate diseases, sore throats, acne, fatigue, sexual problems, allergies have all been successsfully treated by the use of bee pollen.

(Thank you Carlson Wade)

Athletes and coaches use this perfect food for energy, endurance and stamina. According to Harry McCarthy, in *How Bee Pollen Slows Aging,* pollen contains mysterious ingredients which slow down aging and fight killing disease. Pollen boosts an athletes's performance further and much more safely than pep pills.

Start your morning with Lynn's Orange Bee:

In your blender:

8 oz fresh water

1 oz Bee pollen

1 tablespoon of concentrated orange juice

1 capsule of propolis

1 teaspoon honey and ½ cup of fruit. Blend well and enjoy.

Your doctor may hesitate to consider pollen more than just a curiosity in the hall of medicine, but Sen. Tom Harkin's amazing recovery from devastating allergies is attributed to a mix of bee pollen and herbs called Aller Bee-Gone developed by Royden Brown. Mr. Brown recently met with officials at the National Institutes of Health about a clinical trial of his formula to be conducted by the Office of Alternative Medicine. Brown, whose CC Pollen Co. sells Aller Bee-Gone in health food stores at $20 a bottle says his product cures allergies, asthma and other respiratory problems, but says he doesn't know how the formula works.

Pollen supplements are most effective when taken on an empty stomach. The effect is progressive, with the greatest percentage of change coming in about one month.

Pollen supplements are most effective when taken on an empty stomach.

Chapter 14

Powerful Herbal Formulas You Can Make

HERBAL BLENDS OFTEN PRODUCE a broader and more constant effect than individual herbs. If there is a store close to you that sells herbs, you can make the following formulas for yourself. If not, you can get a catalog from a number of mail order companies. Here is one of the best:

Indiana Botanic Gardens

PO BOX 5

Hammond, IN 46325

Blood and Lymph Cleanser

Herbal blends produce a broader effect than individual herbs.

2 oz Echinacea angustifolia

1 oz Smilax ornata

1 oz Arctium lappa

1 oz Berberis vulgaris

3/5 oz Trifolium protense

½ oz Viola odorata

½ oz Petroselinum spp.

½ oz Gallium aparine

½ oz Glycyrrhizae uralensis

½ oz Taraxacum officinale

½ oz Rumex crispus

To make a tincture, combine the herbs with 1 ½ pints of alcohol, such as vodka, brandy, gin or rum, in a container with a tight stopper or lid. Let the mixture stand at room temperature in a dark place for fourteen days, shaking the mixture two or three times daily. Then, after two weeks, let the herbs settle and pour off the tincture. Strain the herbs through a filter or a fine cloth such as muslin, and put the liquids into dark bottles with tight caps.

The adult dose is usually about ½ to one teaspoon.

Antibiotic and Antiviral Mixture

3 oz Echinacea angustifolia

1 ½ oz Hydrastic canadensis

1 oz Arctium lappa

½ oz Commiphora myrrha

Make a tincture as above. The dosage is ½ to one teaspoon, 3 to 6 times a day, depending on the severity of the problem.

Immune System Builder

2 oz Bee propolis

1 oz Eleutherococcus senticosus

1 oz Astragalus membranaceus

1 oz Panax ginseng

1 oz Ligustrum lucidum

½ oz Pyrus malus

½ oz Glycyrrhizae uralensis

Prepare a tincture as shown before and take ½ to one teaspoon three times a day.

These formulas have been given using the botanical origins of the herbs to prevent substitutions based on the familiar names, since many herbs are called by a variety of names. Your supplier will not have any trouble identifying the herbs you want.

Your supplier will not have any trouble identifying the herbs you want.

Chapter 15

Homeopathic Help

YOUR HEALTH FOOD STORE or drugstore carries a number of different brands of homeopathic remedies. Look for one that is heavily advertised. Get the "6x" potency. Potency refers to the number of times that a remedy is repeatedly diluted and shaken or ground. The standard dose is two 6x tablets every two to four hours. Take only one remedy at a time and avoid other medications such as aspirin or laxatives. Do not wash the tablets down with coffee or water. Let them dissolve in your mouth so they can be absorbed directly through the mucous membrane. They are tiny tablets and dissolve easily. Continue taking the remedy until you begin to see improvement, then increase the interval between doses. When improvement is well established, discontinue taking the tablets.

The tiny tablets dissolve easily in your mouth. Continue the remedy until you see improvement.

Choose the best remedy based on the constellation of symptoms rather than what an illness is called.

Aconitum napellus (monkshood). Aconite is useful in the early stages of inflammation or fever and is indicated by the sudden onset of violent symptoms, especially after exposure to dry, cold wind. The patient who needs Aconite is fearful, restless, and thirsty for cold drinks.

Allium cepa (red onion). This remedy will help the person with a beginning cold who looks as if he or she has been peeling onions. There is a frequent sneezing and the eyes stream: a watery discharge irritates the nose. The person may also have laryngitis, with a raw sensation extending to the chest.

Antimonium tartaricum (tartar emetic). This remedy will benefit the person who has bronchitis and a wheezing cough: mucous in the chest makes a rattling, bubbling sound as if the patient were drowning in his or her own secretions. The patient is pale, has a cold sweat, and looks sick.

Apis mellifica (honeybee). This remedy will relieve insect bites, including bee stings, or other rosy red spots with stinging pains.

Arnica montana (leopard's bane). Your first choice for the aftereffects of a fall or overexertion, or injury from a blunt object. The person who needs arnica feels bruised and sore.

Arsenicum album (arsenic). This is the most frequently needed remedy for stomach upsets, vomiting, or diarrhea, especially when caused by food poisoning.

Belladonna (deadly nightshade). The belladonna patient is flushed, hot and restless; symptoms are violent with sudden onset. The person may have sore throat or cough, headache, earache, or fever.

Bryonia alba (white bryonia). Bryonia is called the "grumpy bear" because the person who needs it is irritable and wants to be left alone. Whatever the ailment—fever, headache, sore throat, stomach upset—the patient feels worse from the slightest movement and is very thirsty.

Calcarea phosphorica (phosphate of lime). Calcarea phosphorica aids in the healing of bones and is therefore prescribed for fractures and difficult teething. This remedy also has a beneficial effect on tonsils, neck glands, and schoolchildren's headaches.

Cantharis (Spanish fly). Cantharis relieves the frequent, painful urination that occurs in cystitis. It also alleviates the pain of burns and scalds.

Carbo vegetabilis (vegetable charcoal). Known as the "great reviver," carbo vegetabilis helps the person who is on the verge of collapse or whose vitality is low after an illness.

This remedy will relieve insect bites, including bee stings.

The grief remedy for the person who doesn't recover from an emotional upset such as disappointment or anger.

Chamomilla (German chamomile). The chamomilla child, when teething, is irritable and cranky and just plain "impossible." Chamomilla is helpful for anyone who is oversensitive to pain, particularly when suffering from a toothache.

Ferrum phosphoricum (phosphate of iron). Helps in the early stages of all inflammatory problems, including head colds, earache, cough, pneumonia, bronchitis, pleurisy, and rheumatism.

Gelsemium sempervirens (yellow jasmine). A remedy to consider if the person feels dull, heavy-lidded, complains of aching and chills, is not thirsty, and wants to be left alone. Gelsemium is often needed for flu, head colds, tension headache.

Hepar sulphuris calcareum (calcium sulphide). Helps to localize inflammation, as in bringing a boil to a head. It is useful for certain types of head colds, sore throat, and laryngitis and is the most frequently used remedy for children with croup.

Hypericum perfoliatum (St. John's wort). We call this the "arnica of the nerves" because Hypericum heals injured parts rich in nerves, such as fingertips and toes. It also helps tailbone injuries, even old ones.

Ignatia amara (St. Ignatius bean). Ignatia is the grief remedy for the person who doesn't recover from an emotional upset such as disappointment or anger; patient sighs very frequently.

Ipecacuanha (ipecac root). Ipecac relieves constant nausea with or without vomiting. It also helps to stop a bad nosebleed or bleeding from any part of the body.

Ledum palustre (marsh tea). This is the key remedy for puncture wounds, stings, and bites. Ledum is also helpful in eye injuries and with a sprained ankle.

Magnesia phosphorica (phosphate of magnesia). Some people call this the "homeopathic aspirin." It eases any spasmodic pain that is relieved by warmth, such as leg cramp, menstrual cramps, or colic.

Mercurius visus (quicksilver). This remedy is often indicated for tonsillitis, abscessed ears, boils, and gum disease. The person who needs mercury is sweaty, feels weak and trembling, and is very sensitive to temperature changes.

Nux vomica (poison nut). Sometimes called the "hangover remedy" because it often relieves the person who has overindulged in food or alcohol. Nux vomica also helps the chronic user of laxatives to break the habit.

Phosphorus (phosphorus). Some of the symptoms that indicate a need for phosphorus are laryngitis, a chest cold, and hemorrhaging. Phophorus has a long-lasting effect and should not be repeated often.

Pulsatilla (wind flower). This remedy will help a "ripe" cold with profuse thick, yellow discharge. It will also relieve the person who has an upset stomach from eating too much rich food. The person who needs Pulsatilla loves the open air, is worse from warmth, is not very thirsty, and can't stand fat.

Ruta graveolens (rue). For a shinbone injury, or any injury to the periosteum (bone covering). Ruta graveolens is also useful for sprains. When arnica fails to relieve a bruised, lame feeling resulting from a fall, follow up with ruta.

Spongia tosta (roasted sponge). This remedy's chief indication is a croupy, wheezing cough, and therefore it is prescribed for children during a croup attack.

Sulphur (sublimated sulphur). Homeopaths often prescribe this medication for certain skin diseases that cause dry, itchy skin. Sulphur is more often used in chronic diseases than acute ones.

Veratrum album (white hellebore). A remedy for the distressful time when diarrhea and vomiting occur simultaneously. The patient is in a cold sweat and feels faint.

It relieves the person who has overindulged in food or alcohol.

PART II

New Hearts For Old

"A HEART TRANSPLANT IN A BOTTLE"

Cholesterol Fighters

Nutritional Supplements

Low-Fat Protein

Lecithin, Vitamin E & more

Chelation Therapy

Chapter 16

Cardiovascular Disease

WHAT'S THE RISK of developing cardiovascular disease? The leading cause of death among Americans today is cardiovascular disease.

Cardiovascular disease is:

- Heart Attack
- Stroke
- Embolism
- Aneurysm

Terrifying words and with good reason. Cardiovascular disease (CVD) is responsible for almost as many deaths in the United States as all other causes of death combined.

The leading single cause of death in the United States is heart attack, a particularly dangerous form of CVD, but CVD includes any disease of the heart or blood vessels such as coronary heart disease, rheumatic heart disease, stroke, and hypertension (high blood pressure). Any of these conditions can be extremely serious and potentially life-threatening. Most of us know someone who has fallen victim to one or more of these conditions.

Cardiovascular disease is epidemic in the United States. According to the American Heart Association, over 989,000 Americans die every year from CVD, almost double the number of cancer deaths. Heart attacks accounted for more than fifty percent of the deaths, with strokes running

Heart attacks accounted for more than fifty percent of the cardiovascular disease deaths.

a close second. Every year approximately 350,000 Americans die of heart attacks before they ever reach a hospital.

Those figures are enough to make anyone sit up and take notice but there's another figure that's even more frightening. According to the American Heart Association, more than 63 million Americans have some sort of cardiovascular disease.

Hypertension affects about 55 million adults and over 2 million children in the United States. Many people don't know they have a serious problem and most of them don't have the problem under control even though high blood pressure is easily detectable and usually able to be controlled with diet, supplements or prescription drugs. Education can be your most valuable tool against this killer. If you know the risk factors and are willing to take some simple nutritional steps, you can tilt the scales in your favor and avoid becoming a statistic.

If you know the risk factors and are willing to take some simple nutritional steps, you can tilt the scales in your favor.

Risk Factors in Cardiovascular Disease

By definition, risk factors are habits, conditions, practices, or characteristics that can increase an individual's chances of developing a particular disease. A number of CVD risk factors have been identified. Many can be controlled, reduced, or even eliminated if you decide that your health is in your own hands and take steps to lower your chances of developing CVD.

According to the American Heart Association, these are well-established CVD risk factors:

- Hypertension
- Hypercholesterolemia (high blood pressure)
- Smoking
- Diabetes
- Obesity

In addition to the well-established risk factors, there are the following probable or possible risk factors:

- A family history of CVD
- Type A personality (agressive response to stress)
- Sedentary lifestyle
- Overindulgence in alcohol
- Abuse of drugs

Many CVD risks are closely related to diet and nutrition. The U.S. Department of Agriculture has estimated that a proper diet could reduce CVD deaths by 20 to 25 percent which could mean that over 300,000 people a year could live longer lives. For that reason, many experts emphasize dietary CVD risk factors.

The following dietary factors may be contributory to cardiovascular disease:

- Excessive intake of salt
- Excessive intake of high-fat, high-cholesterol foods
- Insufficient dietary fiber
- Excessive intake of calories
- Low intake of vitamins and minerals

You can improve your diet and nutrition. You can lower your cholesterol count through a low fat diet and useful nutrients, but you will be more inclined to do so if you understand the workings of your heart and circulatory system.

A proper diet could reduce CVD deaths by 20 to 25 percent.

Chapter 17

The Heart And Circulatory System

BELOW ARE DIAGRAMS OF THE HEART and circulatory system. This is basically a closed circular double loop system. The heart pumps oxygen-rich blood first through the major arteries, then through smaller arteries, and finally through even smaller arterioles into tiny capillaries. When the blood reaches the tissues, oxygen and nutrients are absorbed through the capillary walls and exchanged for carbon dioxide and cell wastes.

The heart pumps oxygen-rich blood through the major arteries, then the smaller and smaller ones.

The Circulatory System

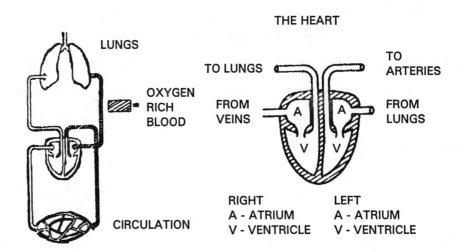

LUNGS

THE HEART

OXYGEN RICH BLOOD

TO LUNGS

TO ARTERIES

FROM VEINS

FROM LUNGS

A   A

V   V

CIRCULATION

RIGHT
A - ATRIUM
V - VENTRICLE

LEFT
A - ATRIUM
V - VENTRICLE

Then the "used" blood, carrying the waste products from the tissues, returns to the heart by passing first out of the capillaries, then through smaller veins, and finally through the major veins. When it reaches the heart, the blood is pumped into the lungs to rid itself of carbon dioxide and pick up a new supply of oxygen. From the lungs, it returns back to the heart to renew its journey.

A number of conditions can obstruct this process, and these conditions are all classified under the heading, Cardiovascular Disease. At the root of most cardiovascular disease, however, lies a condition known as arterio-sclerosis.

Arteriosclerosis at Heart of Most CVD

The most common form of arteriosclerosis, or "hardening arteries," is atherosclerosis. Atherosclerosis occurs when the arteries become thick and hard from a buildup of deposits on their inner walls. These deposits are primarily made up of fat and cholesterol, but may also include fibrin (a clotting material), calcium, and cellular waste.

This buildup on inner artery walls causes the arteries to narrow and lose their ability to expand and contract. The combination of narrowed arteries and loss of elasticity results in reduced blood flow through the arteries to the heart, brain, kidneys, or other parts of the body. Arthero-sclerosis can thus contribute to hypertension, aneurysm, angina, and ischemic heart disease. Even more dangerous, atherosclerosis can lead to heart attack and stroke.

Athero-sclerosis occurs when the arteries become thick and hard from a buildup of deposits and can lead to heart attack and stroke.

Fat And Cholesterol Buildup On Inner Artery Walls

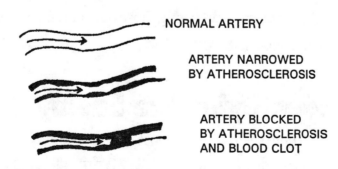

NORMAL ARTERY

ARTERY NARROWED
BY ATHEROSCLEROSIS

ARTERY BLOCKED
BY ATHEROSCLEROSIS
AND BLOOD CLOT

ARROW INDICATES BLOOD FLOW

Sometimes atherosclerotic plaque deposits accumulate enough to block an artery completely. Other times a blood clot forms and attaches itself to a piece of plaque, thereby achieving the same result. If either condition occurs, blood flow through the artery is cut off. When the artery leads to the heart, a heart attack (coronary thrombosis) results. When the blockage occurs in an artery to the brain, a stroke (cerebral thrombosis) results.

Atherosclerosis has been called a silent but deadly disease. It produces no symptoms, and individuals are generally unaware they even have the disease until they are felled by a heart attack, stroke, or other blockage. Unfortunately, for a great number of individuals, sudden death is the first sign of atherosclerosis and CVD.

Too often in modern medicine, attention is based on treatment and not on prevention. Yet with cardiovascular disease, prevention is essential!

The American Heart Association asks Americans to take personal responsibility for their heart. The AHA says:

"A major reduction both in heart attacks and heart death can be achieved only by prevention of heart attacks, not from the treatment of established heart diseases. Almost half of all heart attack deaths occur with the first heart attack and before treatment can be started. Therefore, prevention is a must."

Make the changes that help you protect yourself from CVD. You can't change your parents or a history of diabetes in the family, but you can stop smoking, stop overindulging in alcohol, start eating a diet that's more helpful and you can start taking those nutritional supplements which help your body help itself.

Identifying the Enemy

There seems to be almost universal agreement that cholesterol is the monster that contributes most to CVD. Elevated blood cholesterol levels

With cardiovascular disease, prevention is essential! "Almost half of all heart attack deaths occur with the first heart attack and before treatment can be started."

and other blood fat levels are the most dangerous of all the CVD risk factors. It appears that high blood cholesterol level is contributory to almost half of all the heart attacks in the United States and to a large number of strokes. Therefore, the simple plan to lower your cholesterol level will almost surely reduce your risk of cardiovascular disease.

What Makes A High Blood Cholesterol Level Dangerous?

Cholesterol deposits tend to build up on the inside walls of arteries leading to atherosclerosis. Atherosclerosis is the cause of a majority of CVD. Without this cholesterol buildup, or with it at a minimum, your chances of having a heart attack or a stroke are lowered.

In a nutshell, excess serum cholesterol contributes to atherosclerosis, and atherosclerosis is responsible for most CVD.

How Is Serum Cholesterol Measured?

Serum cholesterol levels are measured as the milligrams of cholesterol per deciliter of blood. Mg/dl is the way it's usually shown when your doctor gets the report. Doctors used to assume that a level from 220 to 300 mg/dl was "normal," but the last decade has seen a change in the safety factor. From world figures, "normal" would be a serum level of from 140 to 180. In the United States, using middle-aged Americans as the norm, the average cholesterol level would be about 200 to 230, so that's our "normal" range.

That doesn't mean that "normal" is good or even acceptable. According to the Framingham Heart Study, in which more than 5,000 residents of Framingham, Massachusetts were monitored for almost 40 years, *nearly half of all heart attacks occurred in persons with cholesterol levels between 200 and 240. Dr. William Castelli, medical director of the study, reported that only one person with cholesterol level of 150 or less had a heart attack.*

> *In a nutshell, excess serum cholesterol contributes to atherosclerosis which is responsible for most CVD.*

Cholesterol is found in every cell in your body . . . naturally.

Read this chart to see how the risk of CVD increases as your cholesterol level rises.

Cholesterol mg/dl	CVD Risk Factor Compared to 180/dl
180 or lower	Safe level, most experts agree
180-200	risk is 25% higher
200-220	risk is 200% higher
220-240	risk is 250% higher
240-280	risk is 300% higher
280-300	risk is 400% higher
300 and up	risk is 500% higher or even more

If all Americans took their hearts in their hands and honestly tried to control their cholesterol levels to arrive at below 200 mg/dl, deaths from CVD could drop anywhere from 30 to 50 percent over the next twenty years. That could add up to a savings of half a million lives a year!

What Is Cholesterol And Where Does It Come From?

First, What Is It?

In its pure form, cholesterol is a white, powdery substance which cannot be seen, tasted or smelled in food.

And Where Is It Found?

It is present in all foods of animal orgin (meat, chicken, eggs, milk and milk products such as cheese, fish, etc.).

It is also found in every cell in your body . . . naturally.

If It's Found Naturally In The Body, Why Is It Dangerous?

A certain amount of cholesterol is needed for the body to function smoothly. It is so important that the liver manufactures more cholesterol every day than we take in from our food. Once a child reaches the age of six months, the liver makes all of the cholesterol we need. After the age of six we don't have to get any cholesterol from food.

Cholesterol is one of a number of fatty substances called lipids which are essential to the well-being of all our bodies. They provide energy, they transport fat-soluble nutrients such as vitamin A, E, and D through the bloodstream to where they're needed, they insulate the body against cold, and they form the sheaths that protect nerve fibers. Lipids also play a part in the manufacture of digestive juices.

So it's not cholesterol that's dangerous.

It's excess cholesterol that causes the trouble!

So All I Have To Do Is Avoid Excess Cholesterol.

Yes and no.

Cholesterol got most of the bad press, but *all* saturated fats are dangerous. Eating cholesterol-rich foods is not the only cause of high blood cholesterol. Saturated fats from butter, lard, beef or pork fat can raise blood cholesterol levels almost twice as fast as dietary cholesterol can.

Not only that, if you take in an excessive amount of saturated fat you'll also raise your triglyceride level. Triglycerides are another type of lipid that can contribute to CVD when present in excessive amounts.

Lowering your cholesterol level also tends to lower your triglyceride level, and lowering your triglyceride level lends to tends to lower your cholesterol level. The American Heart Association recommends that saturated fats should supply no more than 10 percent of your daily calories and that under 30 percent of your total calories should come from fats.

Why Do I Read About "Good" And "Bad" Cholesterol?

High cholesterol is a CVD risk factor. But, the cholesterol total alone is not the whole story. There is HDL (High-Density-Level Cholesterol)

It's not cholesterol that's dangerous, it's excess cholesterol that causes the trouble!

also known as the "good" cholesterol, and LDL (Low-Density-Level) cholesterol, also known as the "bad" cholesterol. There is also another "bad" one known as VLDL or Very-Low-Density Cholesterol.

The relationship betweeen your "good" cholesterol and your "bad" cholesterol in the total cholesterol count is more important than the total cholesterol alone.

The "good" or "bad" depends on how the cholesterol is prepared to be carried in the bloodstream. Cholesterol is a fat and does not mix with water. Your bloodstream is a watery medium so cholesterol must be mixed with water-soluble protein to be carried around the body. This combination of cholesterol (a lipid) and protein is called a lipoprotein.

LDL (Low-Density Lipoprotein) carries cholesterol to be stored in the cells.

That's bad!

HDL (High-Density Lipoprotein) carries cholesterol to the liver to be eliminated from the body.

That's good!

To be considered on the safe side, the ratio between your total cholesterol and your HDL should be not greater than 4:1 (four parts total cholesterol to one part HDL).

For example, if your total cholesterol is 200, your HDL should be no lower than 50. However, if your total cholesterol is 180 or under, don't worry about your HDL. You're probably in better shape than 90 percent of your fellow Americans.

To be safe, the ratio between your total cholesterol and your HDL should be not greater than 4:1.

How Can I Lower My Total Cholesterol and Raise My HDL?

There are a number of steps you can take which will have a good effect on your cholesterol level.

- Limit your consumption of cholesterol to 100 mg for every 1,000 calories you take in.

- Limit your intake of saturated fat.
- Increase your consumption of fiber.
- Engage in a vigorous exercise program with your doctor's approval.
- Lose weight if you are obese.
- Stop smoking if you smoke.
- Reduce your consumption of alcohol.
- Use food supplements which can make your task much easier.

Some foods such as vegetables, fruits, grains, and beans contain little or no saturated fat or cholesterol. Try to substitute them for the cholesterol-laden foods your normally eat. Oat bran, for example, has been shown to lower total cholesterol and increase HDL.

Use this handy chart as a beginning guide to lowering your cholesterol.

Eat more of the cold-water varieties of fish, such as sardines, herring, salmon and tuna.

FOOD	Cholesterol in mg
Fruits, vegetables, grains	0
1 cup skim milk	4
1 cup whole milk	33
1 egg yolk	270
3 ½ ounce serving size, cooked lean fish	65
Chicken, turkey, light meat (no skin)	80
Lean beef	90
Chicken, turkey, dark meat (no skin)	95
Lean lamb	100
Shrimp	150
Beef liver	440
Beef kidney	700

Eat more of the cold-water varieties of fish, such as sardines, herring, salmon and tuna. Not only are they cholesterol-balanced, but they contain an oil named eicosapentaenoic acid (EPA) which can actually help lower total cholesterol and raise the HDL. Much more about fish oil when we get into the use of nutritional supplements.

Saturated Fat, Unsaturated Fat. . . Counting Fat Calories . . .

Too much saturated fat in the diet can lead to CVD, to obesity and even to a disease such as Lupus, an autoimmune disease in which the body actually attacks itself.

Saturated fat is found naturally in animal food but is also produced by a process called hydrogenation. Whenever you see the word hydrogenated on a label, think "saturated fat!"

Most saturated fats are solid at room temperature, but the saturated fats, palm oil and coconut oil obtained from plants, are semi-solid at room temperature.

Polyunsaturated fat is found primarily in plants and tends to lower total cholesterol. However, any oil, when used to excess, can be detrimental to the body, with the possible exception of the oil obtained from cold-water fish.

Monounsaturated fat, which also tends to lower total cholesterol and may also help raise HDL, is found in olive oil and canola oil. Many nutritionists recommend these two oils for cooking.

All vegetable oils are free from cholesterol. Most vegetable oils are high in polyunsaturates, except for palm oil, palm kernel oil and coconut. Those three are high in saturated fats but, because they are inexpensive, they are used by the baking industry. Check the labels before you buy.

Saturated Fat in Common Oils

Coconut oil	92%
Palm kernel oil	88%
Butterfat	88%
Beef fat	52%
Palm oil	51%
Lard	41%
Soybean oil	15%
Olive oil	14%
Canola oil	13%
Corn oil	13%
Safflower oil	9%

Many nutritionists recommend olive oil and canola oil for cooking.

Each gram of fat supplies nine calories.

Each gram of protein or carbohydrate supplies 4 calories. Therefore, ounce for ounce, fat is twice as fattening as either protein or carbohydrates.

How many fat calories do you eat in a day?

Let's say you figure you eat 70 grams of fat in your diet. Multiply 70 by 9 calories and you get 630 calories. Now, let's say you took in 1500 calories that day total. Divide 630 by 1500 and you get 0.42. This means that 42 percent of your total calorie intake came from fat. Unfortunately, that's the average for most Americans.

But it's an unhealthy average!

Current guidelines recommend limiting your fat intake to no more than 30 percent of the total calories in your daily diet. Labels can be misleading when you're counting fat calories, but it doesn't take an Einstein to figure it out.

Find the number of fat calories in a serving of food the easy way:

The label shows the number of grams of fat/serving.

Multiply this number by 9.

Divide that number by the total number of calories in the serving for the percentage of fat calories.

Example:

A hot dog has 120 calories and 11 grams of fat.

Multiply 11 x 9 = 99

Divide 99 by 120 = 0.825

Therefore, the hot dog has 82.5% fat calories.

So, the hot dog is not exactly the kind of meal you want to eat if you're taking care of your heart . . .

In General:

- Consume no more than two tablespoons of polyunsaturated oil a day.
- Consume no more than two tablespoons of margarine a day. Try to get vegetable oil margarine.

Current guidelines recommend limiting your fat intake to no more than 30 percent of the total calories in your daily diet.

- Consume no more than six ounces of meat, fish or poultry daily. Choose lean cuts, trim off all visible fat, serve poultry without the skin, use cold-water fish more often as a replacement for red meat.
- Have two servings of low-fat or non-fat dairy products a day.
- Consume 4 servings of grain a day.
- Have four or more servings of fruits and vegetables daily.

Nutritional supplements can help take you further towards heart health.

Nutritional Supplements for a Healthy Heart

Eating right and exercising goes a long way toward reducing dietary fat and lowering your cholesterol level. Nutritional supplements can help take you further towards heart health. Although you have to have all of the vitamins and all of the minerals, there are particular nutrients which do more than others to protect you against CVD.

Although all vitamins and minerals can be obtained from the food you eat, it may not be possible to obtain these nutrients in the protective higher amounts without the use of food supplements. None of the suggested supplements require a doctor's prescription and all of them can be obtained from your local health food store or pharmacy.

Prevention is the Answer

About one-quarter of all heart attack victims have had no previous symptoms, but CVD is not the inevitable result of aging. Preventive measures can be taken to avoid heart disease. The trick is to start before there are any symptoms.

The following nutrients may look like a formidable listing at first glance but they are usually found combined in one or more multiple formulas. In general, these are the suggested heart-healthy supplements to be used to ward off the complications of cardiovascular disease.

NUTRIENTS	DOSE	COMMENTS
Coenzyme Q-10	50 -100 mg 3 times a day.	Can act against cardiac damage caused by lack of oxygen.
Lecithin	2 capsules with each meal.	Acts as a fat emulsifier. Works best with vitamin E.
Phosphatidyl Choline or Lipotropic Factors	Follow directions on the label.	Helps reduce fat and triglyceride levels in the blood.
L-Carnitine	Up to 500 mg twice a day between meals with 50 mg of vitamin B^1 and 100 mg of vitamin C.	Helps reduce fat and triglyceride levels in the blood. Increases tolerance to stress. Improves oxygen uptake to cardiac muscles.
Odorless Garlic capsules	Take 2 capsules with meals.	Improves heart health and the health of the circulatory system.
Chelated Calcium with Chelated Magnesium	1,500 mg of Calcium and 750 mg of Magnesium daily. Take in divided doses.	Necessary for the proper functioning of the heart muscles.
TMG (Trimethyl-glycine)	50 mg twice a day.	Promotes better use of oxygen by tissues.
MAX EPA Fish Oil or Black Currant Oil or Evening Primrose oil	Follow label instructions. Helps prevent atherosclerosis.	Best sources of essential fatty acids.
Vitamin E	800 -1,000 I.U. daily. Start with 400 I.U.	Helps strengthen the immune system and the heart muscles. Improves circulation. Destroys harmful free radicals.
Selenium	Up to 300 mcg daily. 200 mcg is the usual dose.	Stimulates the immune system. Protects against free radical damage.
L-Taurine	Take with vitamin C and B^6 with juice, not milk.	This amino acid helps correct cardiac arrhythmias when needed.
Vitamin B-Complex	50 mg with meals.	Necessary for correct metabolism of foods.

Helps strengthen the immune system and the heart muscles.

NUTRIENTS	DOSE	COMMENTS
Vitamin C plus Bioflavonoids	1,000 mg three times a day.	Important for heart health.
Vitamin A and/or Beta-Carotene	Up to 25,000 I.U. daily.	Antioxidants that protect against free radical damage.

Plus a good multivitamin/mineral combination containing any of the other supplemental nutrients necessary for the health of your body. For example: zinc has not been included in the specifics for cardiovascular health but zinc takes part in over 800 enzyme reactions and contributes to the immune function. Zinc will be a part of any good multiple vitamin/mineral formula. The same situation applies to iron, copper, and potassium.

Certain nutritional supplements may require additional explanation because, while they are well known to the nutritional community, they have not been given much publicity in the popular press.

L-Carnitine

This nutrient has also been called vitamin Bt although it does not meet the true test of a vitamin, which is that it cannot be manufactured in the body. Carnitine is made in the liver when lysine, methionine, vitamin C, vitamin B^3, vitamin B^6 and the mineral iron are all present in the necessary amounts. Meat and milk products contain carnitine, but these are products you eat in reduced amounts when you are helping your heart. In your body, carnitine is found mostly in the heart and skeletal muscles, and the adrenal gland.

The major role of L-Carnitine is the transportation of fat molecules out of the bloodstream and into the cells where the fat is burned for energy.

The more carnitine present, the more fat that gets taken from the bloodstream and disposed of.

L-Carnitine also helps reduce the risk of CVD by lowering blood triglycerides and by helping to correct heart arrhythmias.

The more carnitine present, the more fat that gets taken from the bloodstream and disposed of.

Fish Oil, MAX EPA, Black Currant Oil, Evening Primrose Oil

Although we are lumping marine fats and plant oils together, it is because they all can improve the blood condition to protect against heart disease. Some people cannot abide eating fish and so lose the protective value that fish oil has to offer. They can't even take fish oil in capsule form because they can "taste" the fish through the capsule or afterwards. That's a pity because fish oil is a wonderful supplement for your heart health. But, if you can't abide fish, then get either the black currant oil or the primrose oil.

Cold-water fish contain EPA (eicosapentaenoic acid) which is required for the production of the prostaglandin-3 family that controls blood clotting, and artery spasms. EPA also improves blood viscosity, lowers cholesterol (especially LDL) and lowers triglycerides. It is in a special class of polyunsaturated fatty acids that biochemists call "Omega-3" fatty acids.

Black currant oil and primrose oil contain a substance called GLA (Gamma Linolenic Acid). Under the best of circumstances, GLA is manufactured in the body from the linoleic acid found in vegetable oils. GLA helps prevent cholesterol from depositing on artery walls. However, the manufacture of this important substance can be interfered with by a deficiency of vitamin B[6], magnesium, or zinc, or a lack of vitamin B[3]. And, in some individuals, the lack of a particular enzyme needed during the GLA manufacturing process also cuts it short.

GLA helps prevent cholesterol from depositing on artery walls.

GLA is found in appreciable amounts in mother's milk, black currant oil and primrose oil. If you prefer, GLA is also available in a prepared supplement form which has concentrated the GLA into a capsule form.

All of these products are available at your health food store or drugstore.

Lipotropics

These are a group of nutrients that have an affinity for fats. Their primary function is to prevent the excessive accumulation of fat in the liver. Lipotropics break fat globules into smaller particle size. This helps the liver metabolize the fatty stores which enables the liver to increase the use of fat as an energy source. Lipotropics also help increase the production of lecithin which lowers the cholesterol content in the bloodstream and helps prevent cholesterol deposits.

Lecithin

Lecithin raises the beneficial HDL and helps lower LDL. This ally against CVD is found naturally in animal and plant tissues and is a source of linoleic acid which the body uses to metabolize cholesterol, triglycerides, and other lipids. Lecithin can help break up fatty cholesterol deposits, reduce total serum cholesterol and lower the LDL, while raising the protective, beneficial HDL component.

Coenzyme Q-10

This nutrient is an essential part of the system which ferries fat out of the blood and into the cells to be burned up for energy.

Some studies have pointed out that there is a deficiency of coenzyme Q-10 found in patients suffering from heart failure, and that the use of this supplement has increased the production of energy in the heart muscles.

Coenzyme Q-10 is found in every cell in your body and is an absolute necessity for energy production, particularly in the cardiovascular system.

Coenzyme Q-10 is found in every cell in your body and is an absolute necessity for energy production, particularly in the cardiovascular system.

Chapter 18

Epidemiological Evidence

NUTRITION IS NO LONGER the sole province of "health nuts." There is a lot of laboratory and clinical evidence about the effectiveness of nutrition as a tool against CVD. Unfortunately, very little of this evidence reaches the public. These are some examples of studies that have been done and published in leading medical and nutritional journals.

Nutr. Res. 3:328-8, 1983

Sable-Amplis, R. et al. Further studies on the cholesterol-lowering effect of apple in humans.

Eating 2 to 3 apples daily for one month was effective in lowering total blood cholesterol levels for 24/30 healthy subjects whose diets were otherwise uncontrolled. Since 2 to 3 grams pectin-in-apple produces the same effect as 6 to 50 gm of purified pectin, other components of apples may also be involved.

Am. J. Clin. Nutr. 34:50-53, 1981

Baig, M.M., Cerda, J.J. Pectin, its interaction with serum lipoproteins.

Grapefruit pectin was found to interact specifically with low-density lipoprotein (LDL), suggesting a biochemical basis by which it may cause the lowering of serum and/or tissue cholesterol levels.

Lancet 1:223-4, 1979

Potter, J.D. et al. Soya saponins and plasma cholesterol.

Eating 2 to 3 apples daily lowered total blood cholesterol levels for 24/30 healthy subjects.

Saponins in plants decrease cholesterol absorption by competing for cholesterol binding sites.

Diabetes 35:604, **1986**

Kamada, T. et al. Dietary sardine oil increases erythrocyte membrane fluidity in diabetic patients.

Sardine oil is rich in eicosapentaenoic acid (EPA is an omega-3 fatty acid) and vitamin E. Supplementation may increase RBC membrane fluidity, thus potentially reducing symptoms due to impaired red cell deformability such as intermittent claudication.

Med. Hypotheses 20:271, **1986**

Bakon, J. Ginger. Inhibition of thromboxane synthetase and stimulation of prostacyclin: relevance for medicine and psychiatry.

Supplementation with ginger may inhibit platelet aggregation (clumping).

Ginger is a potent inhibitor of thromboxane synthetase, as are aspirin and other inhibitors of platelet aggregation. However, ginger is able to raise levels of prostacyclin without a concomitant rise in inflammatory prostaglandins, thus with fewer side effects.

In another study of ginger, reviewed in *Prostagl. Medicine* 13:227, 1984. Srivastrava, K.C. Effects of aqueous extracts of onion, garlic and ginger on platelet aggregation and metabolism of arachidonic acid in the blood vascular system, ginger was found to be more potent than either the garlic or the onion.

Arzneim-Forsch 35:1283-6, **1985**

Schaffler, V.K., Reeh, P.W. Double-blind study of the hypoxia-protective effect of a standardized ginkgo biloba preparation after repeated administration in healthy volunteers.

Supplementation with this substance may relieve the symptoms of peripheral arterial insufficiency.

Sardine oil may reduce symptoms such as intermittent claudication.

There are a number of studies about **garlic**.

- Garlic may reduce cholesterol by inhibiting its synthesis.
  British Med. Journal 291:1391, 1985

- Supplementation may protect against atherogenesis.
  Am. J. Clin. Nutr. 31: 1962,1978

- Garlic and Onions inhibit platelet aggregation by blocking thromboxane synthesis for several hours.
  Lancet, April 7, 1979

- The use of garlic and onion prevented the formation of experimental A S in rabbits.
  Atherosclerosis 26:379-82, 1977

- Aqueous extract of onion and garlic inhibited platelet aggregation induced by several aggregating agents including arachidonate.
  Biomed. Biochim. Acta 43(8/9):S335-S346, 1984

- Fresh garlic completely inhibited platelet aggregation to 5 hydroxytryptamine for 1 to 2 ½ hours after ingestion.
  Lancet 1:776-7, 1981

- 6 healthy subjects took 25 mg of garlic oil daily. After 5 days, platelet aggregation induced by 3 different aggregating agents was completely inhibited.
  Atherosclerosis 30:355, 1978

Biochem. Pharmocol. 34(15):2611-15, 1985
Franconi, F. et al. The protective effect of Taurine on hypoxia.
In isolated guinea-pig heart submitted to hypoxia and subsequent oxygenation, taurine decreased LDH releases and ventricular arrhythmias and increased the recovery of normal electrical and mechanical activity.

Supplementation with this substance may relieve the symptoms of peripheral arterial insufficiency.

Blood cholesterol levels declined 20 percent, and HDL/LDL ratios improved 40 percent.

AM. J. Clin. Nutr. 1810-12, 1979

Malinow, M.R. et al. Alfalfa

Following a diet enriched with 10 tsp. of alfalfa seed powder daily, blood cholesterol levels declined by as much as 20 percent, and HDL/LDL ratios improved by up to 40 percent.

Am. J. Clin. Nutr. 39:917-29, 1984

Story, J.A. et al.

Alfalfa, rich in saponins which are capable of binding to cholesterol and bile salts in the gut to prevent absorption, is capable of reducing cholesterol levels in humans.

Phosphatidyl choline supplementation may not only improve lipoprotein metabolism, but may also cause regression of plaques.

Brit. Journal Exp. Path. 66:35-46, 1985

Hunt, C. et al. Hyperlipoproteinaemia and atherosclerosis in rabbits fed low-level cholesterol and lecithin.

The addition of 3 percent soya lecithin for 3 months successfully restored a healthy distribution of plasma lipoproteins and modified arterial lesions in rabbits with cholesterol-induced atherogenesis.

Phytosterols

Am. J of Clin Nutr. 35:697-700, 1982

Mattson, F.H. et al. Optimizing the effect of plant sterols on cholesterol absorption in man.

300 mg daily (based on beta sitosterol content) immediately before or after meals decreased cholesterol absorption by as much as 64 percent.

Phytosterols are chemical analogs found in plants which can decrease the absorption of cholesterol in the diet, thereby lowering serum cholesterol.

However, according to: *Canadian J. Biochem. Physio.* 36:895, 1958. Beveridge et al.

In research during the late 1950's it was shown that beta sitosterol may reduce serum cholesterol even in the absence of dietary cholesterol. This means that existing serum cholesterol may be lowered by these natural plant substances.

Clin. Ther. 8:537, 1986

Pantothine is the active form of the B-vitamin pantothenic acid. Taking 300 mg 2 to 4 times a day with food can decrease cholesterol and triglyceride levels. It can take 2-4 months to see results and maximal effect can take as long as 4 months.

Glycosaminoglycans

1200 mg three times a day.

Chondroitan sulphate (available in health food stores) is a constituent of acidic glycosaminoglycans found in arterial walls. These substances have anti-coagulant, anti-lipemic, and anti-thrombogenic properties in addition to facilitating wound healing. They appear to form complexes with VLDL and LDL lipoproteins.

Experienta 29:255-7, 1973. Izuka, K., Murata, K.

In a controlled study of 120 CVD patients followed for 6 years, those receiving chondroiton showed fewer abnormal cardiac events than those in a control group. There was also a highly significant difference in the death rate (7 percent of the test group compared to 23 percent of the untreated group).

Coenzyme Q-10

In a dosage of 30 mg, supplementation may reduce anginal episodes and improve cardiac function.

Those receiving chondroiton showed fewer abnormal cardiac events.

Biomed. & Clinical Aspects of Coenzyme Q, Vol. 2. Amsterdam, Elsevier Science Publishers, 1980, p. 247.

In a study, 22 patients showed improvements vs. controls in exercise tolerance.

L-Carnitine

Supplementation may allow the ischemic heart increased energy expenditure before coronary insufficiency develops. It does this by increasing the heart's ability to burn fatty acids.

Int. J. Cardiol. 5:213, 1984

Ferrari, R. et al. The metabolical effects of L-carnitine in angina pectoris.

IV infusions of L-carnitine in 18 coronary artery disease patients improved free fatty acid metabolism and prevented lactate accumulation during atrial pacing, suggesting that L-carnitine may improve myocardial metabolism in such patients.

Bromelain

This is the proteolytic enzyme obtained from pineapples. It is said to inhibit platelet aggregation, relieve angina pectoris and break down arteriosclerotic plaques.

Acta Med. Empirica 5:274-75, 1978

Nieper, H.H. Effect of bromelain on coronary heart disease and angina pectoris.

14 patients with angina pectoris recieved 400-1,000 mg daily with disappearance of symptoms in all patients within 4 to 90 days depending upon the severity of the coronary sclerosis.

It is said to relieve angina pectoris and break down arteriosclerotic plaques.

Chapter 19

Chelation Therapy

WHAT TO DO after a lifetime of the American diet and the deposition of cholesterol plaques in arterial areas which put you at risk for CVD?

A correct diet, with emphasis on a minimum of cholesterol and other fatty intake, should certainly help you in the future, but what about the harm that has already been done to your body? We've read some scientific evidence that says beta sitosterol and phosphatidyl choline may be able to dissolve existing plaques, and now there is the use of chelating agents for the same purpose.

Chelating agents are used to bind with heavy toxic metals such as cadmium, lead, and mercury and excrete them from the body via the natural waste removal systems. They are available in over-the-counter formulations from your health food store for you to use at home. The formulas have been designed to bind with calcium (the basis of many plaques when it accumulates in areas where it does not belong) and help the body excrete that calcium from the body. This has nothing to do with bone calcium and will not effect bones or teeth, just calcium floating in the bloodstream and collecting on arterial walls.

The following chelating agents offer a safe, convenient alternative to people with circulation problems. They can be used to help existing conditions as well as ward off many degenerative illnesses:

Chelating agents can be used to help existing conditions as well as ward off many degenerative illnesses.

- Alfalfa
- Fiber
- Rutin
- Chromium
- Coenzyme Q-10
- Iron chelate
- Kelp

- Selenium
- Calcium chelate
- Magnesium chelate
- Garlic
- Copper chelate
- Zinc chelate

Powerful free radical scavenger.

Supplement	Dose	Comments
Alfalfa	3 times a day with meals	Detoxifies the liver and alkalizes the body. Helps chelate and remove toxic substances from the body.
Coenzyme Q-10	100 mg daily	Improves circulation and lowers blood pressure.
Deod. Garlic	2 daily with each meal	Good chelating agent and detoxifier.
L-cysteine and L-methionine	500 mg twice a day	Source of sulfur. Take with vitamins C and B^6.
Rutin and Apple Pectin	Follow label	Binds heavy metals and removes them from the body via the intestines.
Selenium	200 mcg daily	Powerful free radical scavenger.
Vitamin A	25,000 I.U. daily	Aids in excreting toxic substances.
Vitamin B-Complex	50 mg of each	Protects body.
Vitamin C plus Bioflavonoids in divided doses	Up to 15,000 mg daily	Chelating agent and immune stimulant.
Vitamin E	Up to 600 I.U. daily	Destroys free radicals and limits toxic material.

Also, try to include sulfur-containing legumes, eggs, garlic and onions. Get fiber from oat and wheat bran. Drink eight glasses of water daily.

Intravenous Chelation Therapy

Intravenous therapy is often used to remove calcified, hardened plaque from arterial walls. This will, in turn, improve circulation. This procedure is done only by a physician who understands the concept and is usually used in more serious situations than those which can be helped by oral chelation, although there are clinics which use intravenous chelation therapy to improve the blood flow for anyone who has difficulty with circulation. The patients in these cases may or may not have been diagnosed with CVD in order to obtain chelation therapy.

EDTA (ethylene diamine tetraacetic acid), a synthetic amino acid, is the chelating agent. It is administered intravenously to treat such ailments as high blood pressure and heart disease. EDTA is slowly released into the bloodstream over a two to four hour period during which the patient usually reads a book or converses with other people getting the same therapy. As the EDTA travels around the body through the arteries, it binds with the calcium that has been deposited along the walls and excretes it from the body through the kidneys.

EDTA is a strong chelating substance and also attracts lead, strontium and other divalent metals for removal. This procedure is controversial and has as many doctors against it as for it. However, when done correctly, it has not been found to be harmful. Therefore, it should only be done under the supervision of a qualified physician.

If you are interested in chelation intravenous therapy, you can contact these groups for information about a doctor in your area:

The American College of Advancement in Medicine
23121 Verdugo Drive, Suite 204
Laguna Hills, CA 92653
(714) 583-7666

The American Board of Chelation Therapy
70 West Huron Street
Chicago, IL 60610
(312) 787-2228

It also attracts lead, strontium and other metals for removal.